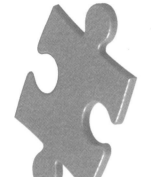

Nephrology Nursing Scope and Standards of Practice

7th Edition

Editor

Norma J. Gomez, MBA, MSN, RN, CNN

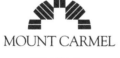

MOUNT CARMEL

A MEMBER OF ✛ TRINITY HEALTH

THERESE PACE,
MSN, RN, CCRN
Clinical Educator
SIMCU & 3-South

(614) 234-7716
tpace@mchs.com

6001 East Broad Street · Columbus, Ohio 43213-1502
mountcarmelhealth.com

Amer

www.annanurse.org

Nephrology Nursing Scope and Standards of Practice, 7th Edition
Copyright © 2011 American Nephrology Nurses' Association

Editor
Norma J. Gomez

Publication Management
Anthony J. Jannetti, Inc.
East Holly Avenue/Box 56, Pitman, New Jersey 08071-0056

Managing Editor: Claudia Cuddy
Editorial Assistant: Katie R. Brownlow
Layout Design and Production: Claudia Cuddy
Cover Design: Darin Peters
Design Consultant: Jack M. Bryant
Copy Editor: Claudia Cuddy
Proofreader: Katie R. Brownlow

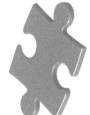

ANNA National Office Staff
Executive Director: Michael Cunningham
Director of Membership Services: Lou Ann Leary
Manager, Chapter Services: Janet Betts
Coordinator, Education Services: Wendy Hankin
Coordinator, Membership Services: Julie Atkinson
Program Manager: Celess Tyrell
Executive Assistant and Marketing Manager, Advertising: Susan Iannelli
Fulfillment Coordinator: Kathi Hacker
Director of Education Services: Sally Russell
Director of Marketing: Tom Greene
Managing Editor, *Nephrology Nursing Journal*: Carol Ford
Editorial Coordinator, *Nephrology Nursing Journal*: Joe Tonzelli
Managing Editor, *ANNA Update* & *ANNA E-News*, Web Editor: Kathleen Thomas
Director, Public Relations and Association Marketing Services: Janet D'Alesandro
Public Relations Specialist: Linda Alexander
Director, Electronic Publishing: Todd Lockhart
Director, Creative Design and Production: Jack M. Bryant
Creative Designers: Darin Peters, Bob Taylor
Conference Manager: Jeri Hendrie
Conference Coordinator: Cary Fredericks
Vice President, Fulfillment and Information Services: Rae Ann Cummings
Director, Fulfillment and Information Services: Robert McIlvaine
Comptroller: Patti Fortney
Bookkeeper: Jennifer Dennison
CEO Anthony J. Jannetti, Inc.: Tony Jannetti

ANNA Disclaimer
The *Nephrology Nursing Scope and Standards of Practice* is designed to provide information and assist decision making. The Nephrology Nursing Process of Care statements within this document are not intended to define a care guideline and should not be construed as one. Neither should they be interpreted as prescribing an exclusive course of management. If a clinician is looking for prescriptive information regarding the management of the patient with kidney disease, he or she should examine other literature with the most current evidence-based information. Each nurse is responsible for evaluating the appropriateness for the particular clinical situation.

American Nephrology Nurses' Association, East Holly Avenue/Box 56, Pitman, New Jersey 08071-0056
Web site: www.annanurse.org ■ E-mail: anna@ajj.com ■ Phone: 888-600-2662

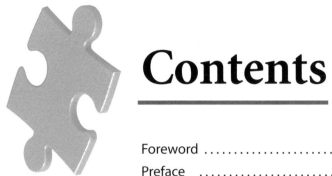

Contents

1 Nephrology Nursing Scope of Practice 1

2 Nephrology Nursing Standards of Practice 15

3   How to Use the Standards in Practice 37

4   Nephrology Nursing Process of Care 57

Continued

Continued

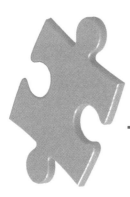

Foreword

The first edition of these standards was published in 1977. Since then, ANNA has periodically revised and updated these standards to address changes in practice and to incorporate evidence-based guidelines as those have been developed.

The next several years will be marked by the transformation of our health care system. The changes will include major ones in nephrology. Standards of practice are a set of guidelines for providing high-quality nursing care. Such guidelines help assure patients are receiving high-quality care. Guidelines are based on the best available evidence, and they serve as a clinical, quality, and if necessary, a legal reference, when questions arise regarding quality of care.

The ANNA Board of Directors and I commend Editor and Project Director Norma Gomez, MBA, MSN, RN, CNN, and each contributor for their efforts in updating this seventh edition. We hope this publication will be valuable to you as you provide quality care.

Donna Painter, MS, RN, CNN
ANNA President, 2010–2011

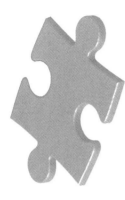

Preface

The recently revised American Nurses Association's (ANA) *Nursing: Scope and Standards of Practice* (2010) provides both a broad foundation for defining nursing practice and a comprehensive guide for the evaluation of that practice. There are several changes in the 2010 edition of the standards. The most evident is the change from *measurement criteria* to *competencies*. A second change is the incorporation of the *advanced practice registered nurse* into the overall standards.

The American Nephrology Nurses' Association (ANNA) *Nephrology Nursing Scope and Standards of Practice,* 7th edition, has been refined for nephrology nursing and presents a similar approach as the ANA standards. An editor and workgroup were identified to revise the current nephrology nursing scope, standards of practice, and guidelines for care. The workgroup developed a project plan and contacted experts in the field. The Special Interest Groups (SIGs) were involved in the review process. Draft revisions were posted on the ANNA website for member response. The board of directors reviewed the definition of nephrology nursing, the scope of practice, and the nephrology nursing standards prior to submitting to ANA for endorsement.

The 7th edition has expanded to incorporate an introduction to nephrology nursing. Incidentally, the information used in this section is from the ANNA application to ANA for recognition of nephrology nursing as a specialty in nursing. The application was authored by Caroline Counts, MSN, RN, CNN, president of ANNA, 2003–2004, and Beth Ulrich, EdD, RN, CHE, president of ANNA, 1984–1985, and editor of *Nephrology Nursing Journal.* Special thanks must be given to their dedication to nephrology nursing. Also included in the introduction of the ANNA standards is a definition of nephrology nursing and an updated scope of practice statement. Another addition is the section of examples on how to use the standards in clinical practice. A short vignette provides the reader with an overview of a situation that requires intervention by the nephrology nurse. Samples of tools that incorporate the standards into the various situations are included.

The section on *nephrology nursing process of care for the patient with kidney disease* provides the nephrology nurse with measurable patient outcomes, nursing assessment, nursing interventions, and patient teaching. A glossary has been added to aid with the understanding of terms used in all the sections. Examples of the new terms used in this edition include *kidney replacement therapies* (KRT) in place of *renal replacement therapies* (RRT) and *healthcare consumer* used synonymously with *patient*. The term *family* relates to family of origin or significant others as identified by the patient.

In brief, the *Nephrology Nursing Scope and Standards of Practice* provides nephrology nursing with a method of defining the scope of its practice and a conduit for the evaluation of that practice. Moreover, this document serves as a guide in the identification of the nephrology nurse's responsibilities to their profession, their colleagues, and the healthcare consumer.

Norma J. Gomez, MBA, MSN, RN, CNN
Editor

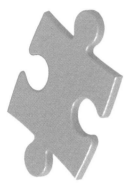

Acknowledgments

Sincere appreciation is extended to the ANNA Board of Directors (2010-2011) for their commitment to quality patient care.

Special acknowledgment goes to the editors, contributors, and reviewers of previous editions of ANNA's Standards of Clinical Practice:

1977	*Standards of Clinical Practice for the Nephrology Patient*
1982	*Nephrology Nursing Standards of Clinical Practice*
1988	*ANNA Standards of Clinical Practice for Nephrology Nursing*
1993	*Standards of Clinical Practice for Nephrology Nursing*
1999	*Standards and Guidelines of Clinical Practice for Nephrology Nursing*
2005	*Nephrology Nursing Standards of Practice and Guidelines for Care*

Thank you to Beth Ulrich and Caroline Counts for their work on the ANA application for specialty practice recognition.

Special appreciation goes to Claudia Cuddy, Managing Editor, for her help in making this edition a reality.

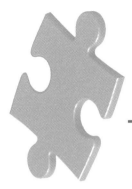

Contributors

Deb Castner, MSN, RN, APNc, CNN
Hazel Dennison, DNP, RN, APNc, CPHQ
Lesley Dinwiddie, MSN, RN, FNP, CNN
Debra Hain, DNS, RN, GNP-BC
Diana Hlebovy, BSN, RN, CHN, CNN
Eileen Peacock, MSN, RN, CNN, CIC, CPHQ, CLN

Focus Group

Sharon Burbage, RN, CNN
Debbie Heinrich, RN, CNN
Sara Kennedy, BSN, RN, CNN
Corinna King, RN, CNN
Melinda Martin-Lester, BA, RN, CNN, CHC
Debra McDillon, MSN, RN, CNN
Holly McFarland, MSN, RN, CNN
B. Sandy Micholics, RN, CNN
Sylvia Moe, BSN, RN, CNN
Leonor Ponferrada, BSN, RN, CNN
Karen Robbins, MS, RN, CNN
Susie Soares-Phillips, RN, CNN
Caroline Steward, ASN, RN, APN, CCRN, CNN
Diane Truchot, MSN, RN, FNP-BC

*Thank you to our Special Interest Groups
for their review.*

SIGS

Acute Care
Administration
Advanced Practice
Chronic Kidney Disease
Hemodialysis
Transplant

Reviewers

Jeffrey Albaugh, PhD, APRN, CUCNS
Diane Alexander, MS, BSN, RN, CNN
Gail Alexander, MSN, RN, CNN
Deborah Bakken, RN, CNN
LaVonne Burrows, APRN, BC, CNN
Sally Burrows-Hudson, MS, RN, CNN
Christine Ceccarelli, PhD, MBA, RN
Christine Corbett, MSN, RN, APRN, FNP-BC
Sue Fallone, RN, CNS, CNN
Jonathan Flores, BSN, RN
Glenda Harbert, ADN, RN, CNN, CPHQ
Liz Howard, RN, CNN
Judy Kaufman, BSN, RN, CNN
Frank Keller, MSN, RN
Carol Kinzner, MSN, GNP-BC, CNN-NP
Mary Rose Kott, MS, RN, ANP, CNN
Deuzimar Kulawik, MSN, RN
Eileen Lischer, MA, BSN, RN
Alice Luehr, BA, RN, CNN
Mark Meier, MSW, LICSW
Sylvia Moe, BSN, RN, CNN
Denise Murcek, MSN, APRN, NP-C, CNN
Linda Myers, BSN, RN, CNN, HP
Clara D. Neyhart, BSN, RN, CNN
Kathy P. Parker, PhD, RN, FAAN
Sonya Peterson, MSN, RN, CNN
Leonor P. Ponferrada, BSN, RN, CNN
Christy Price Rabetoy, RN, CNN, NP
Timothy Ray, MSN, ND, CNP, CNN
Troy Russell, MSN, ACNP-BC, CNN-NP
Karen Schardin, BSN, RN, CNN
Dori Schatell, MS
Patty Spina, BSN, RN, CCRN
Susan VanBuskirk, BSN, RN, CNN
Patricia Weiskittel, MSN, CNN, ACNP
Karen Wiesen, MS, RD, LD
Helen F. Williams, MSN, RN, CNN
Candace Wright, BSN, RN, CNN

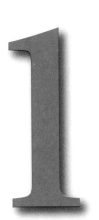

Nephrology Nursing Scope of Practice

Definition of Nephrology Nursing

Nephrology nursing is a specialty practice addressing the protection, promotion, and optimization of the health and well-being of individuals with kidney disease. These goals are achieved through the prevention and treatment of illness and injury, and the alleviation of suffering through patient, family, and community advocacy.

Scope of Practice for Nephrology Nursing

The purpose of the scope of practice for nephrology nursing is to describe, for the public and the profession, the nature of this specialty's nursing practice. The specialty's scope is derived from the scope of nursing practice as defined by the American Nurses Association (2010b) and builds on the previous versions published by the American Nephrology Nurses' Association (ANNA).

Nephrology nursing encompasses the primary, secondary, and tertiary care of individuals with potential and progressive chronic kidney disease (CKD), end-stage renal disease (ESRD), acute kidney injury (AKI), and other health care conditions requiring nephrologic intervention. Nephrology nursing practice spans the continuum of care for patients with kidney disease. Nephrology nurses provide care to neonatal, pediatric, adult, and geriatric individuals from a variety of ethnic groups. The nursing care may be extremely complex as this patient population may have various comorbid conditions including cardiovascular disease, diabetes, hypertension, infectious disease, and/or mineral and bone disease. In addition, many face psychosocial issues.

The term *kidney replacement therapies* (KRT) is being used in the nephrology community in place of the older term *renal replacement therapies* (RRT). These terms identify all therapies used to treat kidney disease including dialysis, transplantation, and palliative care. Throughout this publication, the terms *healthcare consumer* and *patient* will be used interchangeably. *Healthcare consumer* is defined as the patient, person, client, family, group, community, or population who is the focus of attention and to whom the registered nurse is providing services as sanctioned by the state regulatory bodies (ANA, 2010b). The term *family* relates to the family origin or significant others as identified by the patient. The ANA standards use the term *interprofessional* defined as reliant on the overlapping knowledge, skills, and abilities of each professional team member. However, the ANNA work group determined to continue the usage of *interdisciplinary* as reflected in the Centers for Medicare and Medicaid Services (CMS) Conditions for Coverage (CfCs) (CMS, 2008).

Overview of the Scope of Practice for Nephrology Nursing

The recognition of kidney disease, acute and chronic, as a major health problem has led to the development of nephrology nursing as a specialty. The practice of nephrology nursing encompasses the roles of direct caregiver, educator, coordinator, consultant, administrator, and researcher. The practice extends to all care delivery settings in which patients experiencing, or at risk for developing, chronic kidney disease (CKD) stages 1 through 5, receive health care, education, and counseling for kidney disease prevention, diagnosis, progression, and treatment.

Optimal individual functioning and family functioning throughout all phases of disease management are the primary goals of nephrology nursing. The nephrology nurse achieves these primary goals by diagnosing and treating human responses exhibited by individuals and families with kidney disease diagnoses or who are at risk for developing CKD. These human responses include, but are not limited to, physical symptoms, functional limitations, psychosocial disruptions, and knowledge needs.

Treatment of these responses involves health promotion and disease prevention counseling, health maintenance education, psychosocial support to build or sustain coping capacity, education to encourage active participation in decision making and self-care, restorative physical care to manage disease and treatment-related symptoms, and the delivery of kidney-replacement therapies including transplantation.

The focus of the nephrology nurse is the patient, an entity that can include individuals, families, groups, and communities. Nephrology nurses manage care to meet the special needs of the patient with kidney disease to maximize independence and quality of life.

Nephrology nursing practice occurs throughout the patient's life span, along a continuum of care and across delivery settings. Care requirements extend beyond kidney disease to address acute and/or chronic causative disease processes, as well as subsequent comorbid complications. The nature of this nursing care spans the spectrum from preventive and acute through replacement therapies and rehabilitation, as well as palliative, supportive care. Nephrology nursing may be provided in a variety of settings that include, but are not limited to, inpatient, outpatient, freestanding clinics, and home care.

All nephrology nurses are legally, ethically, and morally responsible for practicing in accordance with recognized standards of professional nursing practice, professional performance, the recognized professional code of ethics, and specialty certification.

As illustrated in Figure 1.1, the foundation for nephrology nursing underpins state nurse

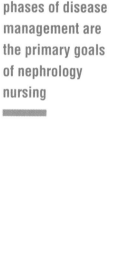

Optimal individual functioning and family functioning throughout all phases of disease management are the primary goals of nephrology nursing

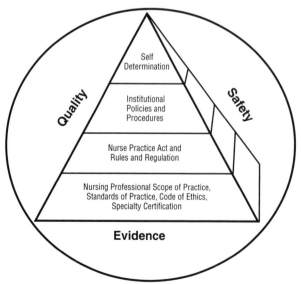

Figure 1.1
Model of Professional Nursing Practice Regulation
(Styles et al., 2008)

© 2010 by American Nurses Association. Redrawn with permission. All rights reserved.

practice acts and institutional policies and procedures. The apex of this model of professional responsibility is achieved with the individual nephrology nurse's assumption of personal accountability for continuing education and professional experience over and above the basic requirements for professional nephrology nursing.

General Nephrology Nursing Practice

In addition to basic educational preparation to function as a registered nurse, nephrology nursing practice at the generalist level requires a specific knowledge base and demonstrated clinical expertise in kidney disease care.

The nephrology nurse coordinates care in collaboration with other care providers and health team members to plan and provide required care as effectively as possible. The nephrology nurse acts as a patient guide and advocate, assisting the patient in seeking information, assuring that the patient has the opportunity for informed consent for treatment decisions, and promoting the maximal level of patient-desired independence. The nephrology nurse may also function in the role as a nurse manager to assure patient safety and the delivery of appropriate care.

The nephrology nurse is accountable for delivering care within the framework of the nursing process. The nephrology nurse uses assessment findings to formulate nursing diagnoses and prioritize problems according to patient need. The nephrology nurse engages the patient in mutual goal setting and collaboration in developing a plan of care directed toward achieving identified goals. The effectiveness of the plan of care in goal achievement is evaluated through patient outcomes.

The nephrology nurse actively participates in professional role development activities including continuing education, quality assessment and improvement, and the review and clinical application of research findings to assure evidence-based practice. The nephrology nurse develops ethically sound practice and confronts ethical challenges through application of the *Nephrology Nursing Scope and Standards of Practice*.

Advanced Practice in Nephrology Nursing

Advanced practice in nephrology nursing requires substantial analytical knowledge in nephrology nursing, and the application and advancement of that knowledge in providing expert care to individuals diagnosed with kidney disease, their families, and the community at large. This advanced practice may include the roles of primary care provider, coordinator, consultant, educator, researcher, and administrator.

Consistent with ANA's *Nursing's Social Policy Statement* and *Consensus Model for APRN Regulation: Licensure, Accreditation, Certificaton & Education* (APRN Consensus Work Group, 2008), the minimum requirements for an advanced practice registered nurse (APRN) with specialization in nephrology are graduate level preparation and certification in an APRN role and at least one population focus, including family/individual across the lifespan, adult-gerontology, neonatal, pediatrics, women's health/gender related, and/or psychiatric-mental health. The APRN with a specialty in nephrology has additional didactic and clinical course work and experiences in that area.

The advanced practice registered nurse prescribes in accordance to state and federal regulations. The advanced practice registered nurse uses specific pharmacologic knowledge and experience to adjust medications as indicated for the patient with kidney disease. The advanced practice registered nurse participates in the development and assessment of medication protocols.

Nephrology nurses practicing at the advanced level must be able to assess, diagnose, theorize, and analyze complex clinical and nonclinical problems related to the actual or potential diagnosis of kidney disease. In addition, *advanced practice* denotes the ability to consider a wide range of theory and research relevant to understanding kidney disease-related problems

Roles of the APRN:

- primary care provider
- care coordinator
- consultant
- educator
- researcher
- administrator

and the ability to select and justify the application of the most meaningful theory or research to assist in problem solving. The advanced practice registered nurse contributes knowledge of nephrology nursing research to interdisciplinary workgroups to assure evidence-based guidelines are incorporated into nephrology nursing practice. The advanced practice registered nurse may serve as the *primary care provider* to an individual diagnosed with kidney disease, their family, and the community.

As a *care coordinator*, the role involves the expert use of the application of change process with the interdisciplinary nephrology care team to determine and achieve realistic health care goals for the particular individual, the family, and/or an entire community, while guiding the patient through the health care system. The *consultant* role in advanced nephrology nursing practice involves providing expert advice about nephrology to colleagues, allied health personnel, and healthcare consumers. The *educator* role is exemplified by the assessment of learning needs, design, implementation, and evaluation of educational activities. The role of the *researcher* requires skills in the use of the research process, which includes the ability to identify current researchable problems in nephrology nursing, collaborate in research, and evaluate and implement research findings that affect patient care or nephrology nursing. The *administrative* role involves use of the managerial process to promote a practice environment that reduces environmental health risks for the nephrology nurse, the patient, and the public.

Nephrology advanced nursing practice is best defined as *expert competency and leadership in the provision of care to individuals with an actual or potential diagnosis of kidney disease.*

> **Nursing encompasses the sciences, the arts, and philosophies in its practice**

Theoretical Foundation of Nursing

Nephrology nurses, especially those working in outpatient facilities, need to remain connected to professional nursing and its theoretical foundatons. In the majority of outpatient dialysis settings, there is no infrastructure for nursing support. This section provides an overview of the profession of nursing. Nursing focuses on the promotion and maintenance of health and the prevention or resolution of disease, illness, or disability. The nursing needs of human beings are identified from a holistic perspective and are met within the context of a culturally sensitive, caring interpersonal relationship (ANA, 2010b).

Science is concerned with causality (i.e., cause and effect). In contrast, philosophy is concerned with the purpose of human life, the nature of the being, and the theory and limits of knowledge. Nursing encompasses the sciences, the arts, and philosophies in its practice.

The science of nursing is based on a critical thinking framework known as the nursing process that comprises assessment, diagnosis, outcomes identification, planning, implementation, and evaluation. These steps serve as the foundation of clinical decision making and are used to provide evidence-based practice.

The art of nursing is based on a framework of caring and respect for human dignity. A compassionate approach to patient care carries an obligation to provide that care competently. Competent care is provided and accomplished through independent practice and collaborative partnerships. Collaboration may be with other colleagues or the individuals seeking support or assistance with their health care needs. Central to the nursing practice is the art of caring, which is represented by the interpersonal relationship that the nurse establishes with the patient.

Nursing Theories

Nephrology nursing practice should be grounded in nursing theory. Nursing theory provides structure and organization to nursing knowledge, and a systematic means of collecting data to describe, explain, and predict nursing practice. Nursing theory should be used in the development of policies and procedures, training and education, clinical information systems, quality improvement programs, and professional development programs.

It is sometimes difficult to decide when, where, and how to apply nursing theories. Nursing theories based on human needs, nursing process, caring, competency, and self-care may be adapted easily to nephrology nursing. Four of the nursing theorists and brief synopses of their theories are discussed below.

Jean Watson's model of human care focuses on the interpersonal relationship between the nurse and patient. Watson highlights the role of the nurse in defining the patient as a unique human being and emphasizes the importance of the connections between the nurse and patient. Watson's transpersonal caring–healing framework describes the following essential concepts:

- The whole caring–healing consciousness is contained within a single caring moment.
- The one caring and the one being cared for are interconnected.
- Human caring and healing processes (or the noncaring, nonhealing consciousness of the nurse) are communicated to the one being cared for.

Madeline Leininger's theory of cultural care diversity and universality addresses care for people from a broad range of cultures, and comprises five theoretical assumptions on caring:

- Care is essential for human growth and survival, and to face death.
- There can be no curing without caring.
- Expressions of care vary among all cultures of the world.
- Therapeutic nursing care can only occur when cultural care values, expressions, or practices are known and used explicitly.
- Nursing is a transcultural care profession and discipline.

Dorothea Orem's theory of self-care deficit nursing theory (SCDNT) is based on the belief that humans require continuous and deliberate inputs into themselves and interaction with their environment to remain alive and to function. The theory purports five methods of helping:

- Acting for and doing for others
- Guiding others
- Supporting another
- Providing an environment promoting personal development in relation to meet future demands
- Teaching another

The dialysis arena is one area of nursing practice in which the application of this theory would be appropriate because it is crucial for patients to be actively involved in self-care (Simmons, 2009).

The **American Association of Critical-Care Nurses** (AACN) **synergy theory** links clinical practice to patient outcomes. The needs or characteristics of the patient and families influence and drive the characteristics or competencies of the nurse. When nurse competencies stem from patient needs and the characteristics of the nurse and patient synergize, optimal patient outcomes can result (AACN Certification Corporation, 2003).

Several assumptions guide the AACN synergy model for patient care. These assumptions must be viewed in context:

- Patients are biological, psychological, social, and spiritual entities who present at a particular developmental stage. The whole patient (body, mind, and spirit) must be considered.
- The patient, family, and community all contribute to providing a context for the nurse–patient relationship.
- Patients can be described by a number of characteristics. All characteristics are connected and contribute to each other. Characteristics cannot be looked at in isolation.

The needs or characteristics of the patient and families influence and drive the characteristics or competencies of the nurse

- Similarly, nurses can be described on a number of dimensions. The interrelated dimensions paint a profile of the nurse.
- A goal of nursing is to restore a patient to an optimal level of wellness as defined by the patient. Death can be an acceptable outcome, in which the goal of nursing care is to move a patient toward a peaceful death.

Evolution of Nephrology Nursing

As early as 1915, nursing literature mentions the care of patients with kidney disease. In the early stages of nephrology nursing, most nursing authors focused on the physical care of these patients, including:

- Recording intake and output
- Controlling the diet
- Maintaining elimination of wastes through the gastrointestinal tract
- Providing sufficient rest
- Preventing infection
- Decreasing muscle activity to minimize the production of metabolic wastes
- Keeping the patient comfortable

The Artificial Kidney (Coleman & Merrill, 1952) was the first article published in the nursing literature to describe the role of the nurse in dialysis. In 1960, the arteriovenous shunt was developed, enabling the long-term treatment of kidney failure with hemodialysis. As the number of patients on hemodialysis increased and the techniques advanced, it was no longer feasible or necessary for physicians to remain at the bedside during the treatments. Nurses assumed responsibility for the majority of hemodialysis procedures (Hoffart, 1989).

Nurses also began working in peritoneal dialysis. They had to initiate, maintain, and monitor the patient and the therapy. This involved recording the intake and output, handling drainage problems, and keeping the patient safe. Infection control and the prevention of peritonitis were major concerns (Fulton & Cameron, 1989; Hoffart, 1989).

Throughout history the possibility of transplanting organs and tissues from one body to another has been intriguing. More than 50 years have passed since the first long-term successful kidney transplant was performed. Nephrology nurses have been involved in every phase of the procedure. From organ procurement to the postoperative phase, nephrology nurses are active members of the interdisciplinary team. The early work of nephrology nurses caring for patients with kidney transplants greatly contributed to the development of other transplant nursing programs.

Nephrology nursing as a specialty began in earnest as kidney dialysis and transplant units were established throughout the United States. These equipment-dependent methods of treatment threatened to dehumanize patients and take away their control. The patients and their families felt the stress of being dependent on a dialysis machine, the stress of financial concerns, the stress of following a strict medical regimen, and the stress resulting from changes in lifestyle (Hoffart, 1989). Nephrology nurses work to personalize the experience and to provide holistic care.

Nephrology Nursing Process

Nephrology nurses use the nursing process in providing care to patients with kidney disease. The nursing process comprises assessment, diagnosis, outcomes identification, planning, implementation, and evaluation. Each phase of the nursing process interacts with and is influenced by the other phases.

> A goal of nursing is to restore a patient to an optimal level of wellness as defined by the patient

Assessment

The nephrology registered nurse collects comprehensive data pertinent to the healthcare consumer's health and/or the situation.

Diagnosis

The nephrology registered nurse analyzes the assessment data to determine the diagnoses or the issues.

Outcomes Identification

The nephrology registered nurse identifies expected outcomes for a plan individualized to the healthcare consumer or the situation.

Planning

The nephrology registered nurse develops a plan that prescribes strategies and alternatives to attain expected outcomes.

Implementation

The nephrology registered nurse implements the identified plan, coordinates care delivery, and employs strategies to promote health and a safe environment. The advanced practice registered nurse specializing in nephrology provides consultation to influence the identified plan, enhance the abilities of others, and effect change. The advanced practice registered nurse performs and reviews procedures, makes referrals, uses prescriptive authority, and provides treatments and therapies in accordance with state and federal laws and regulations.

Evaluation

The nephrology registered nurse evaluates progress toward attainment of outcomes.

> Wherever they practice, nephrology nurses use critical thinking to respond to the needs of patients with kidney disease

Differentiated Areas of Nephrology Nursing Practice

Nephrology nurses work in a variety of multidisciplinary and interdisciplinary environments. The majority of nephrology nursing practice focuses on the patient population with identified kidney disease. Nephrology nurses also practice within the community in the prevention and identification of kidney disease. Patient care is provided through a team approach involving nurses, patient care technicians, machine technicians, social workers, dietitians, physicians, and medical directors. The nephrology registered nurse provides clinical supervision of the licensed practical/vocational nurse (LPN/LVN) and patient care technicians (PCT) in accordance with state practice acts and the Centers for Medicare and Medicaid Services (CMS) Conditions for Coverage (CfCs) regulations (CMS, 2008). Wherever they practice, nephrology nurses use critical thinking to respond to the needs of patients with kidney disease. They are mindful of resource utilization through the implementation of strategies and interventions that provide optimal outcomes most appropriate to the healthcare consumer or situation.

The practice of nephrology nursing may include, but is not limited to, those practices listed below.

Staff nurse, hospital or outpatient settings. The nephrology nurse may work in the inpatient or outpatient setting. Inpatient includes hospital units dealing with patients with acute kidney injury (AKI), kidney disease, and transplant. The outpatient setting may include stand-alone facilities, physician offices, and CKD clinics. These nephrology nurses focus in the areas of hemodialysis, peritoneal dialysis, transplant, organ recovery, quality management, infectious diseases, case management, CKD, and diabetic teaching.

Chronic kidney disease management. One of the nephrology nurse's primary roles is to educate patients with kidney disease about their disease, prognoses, and treatment options. Nephrology nurses also guide patients and their families on strategies and interventions to prevent the progression of their kidney disease.

Advanced practice nursing. The advanced practice registered nurse (APRN) provides care for patients along the continuum of kidney disease and in all treatment modalities. APRNs are used in the inpatient and outpatient settings with the APRN functioning as clinicians, consultants, educators, and researchers.

Case management. The nephrology nurse case manager oversees the quality, outcome, and cost of patient care. Patient advocacy and continuity of care are two vital components of this role.

Education. Many opportunities are available for nurses in nephrology education. The majority of nephrology education is provided by nephrology nurse educators in dialysis facilities. This role is an integral part of staff training and development. The nephrology nurse educator provides patient education using diversified training strategies. Some of the tools available to the nurse educator are interactive training programs, gaming, and Internet sites. The nephrology nurse educator is a valuable resource for facility and hospital staff, nurses from other disciplines, patient educators, and community outreach. In the academic setting, nephrology nurse educators may choose to teach basic nursing, master's, or doctoral level programs.

Management. Nephrology nurses with leadership skills are ideal for the many management and administrative positions in both the inpatient and outpatient settings. Responsibilities of this role may include budgetary compliance, inventory control, regulatory compliance, contract negotiation, oversight of staff education and competency programs, patient education and training, and continuous quality improvement programs.

Research. As nephrology nursing focuses on evidence-based practice, the researcher's role has expanded.

Corporate/government. Corporate employers include manufacturers and distributors of dialysis equipment and related products, as well as pharmaceutical companies. Nephrology nurses may be clinical nurse specialists or directly involved in the development of equipment and products. In government settings, nurses are involved on the local, state, and federal levels.

Nursing informatics. Nursing informatics, a relatively new area, requires nephrology nursing contributions. In this role, the nephrology nurse is responsible for managing and communicating data as well as the development and implementation of electronic medical record systems using information technology guidelines.

Miscellaneous areas for nephrology nursing contribution include legislation, professional associations, home health, and hospice nursing.

There are increasing requirements from regulatory agencies to report "in-time" data on the nephrology workforce. This presents a problem to the specialty in the ability to obtain current workforce data. The time involved and the financial impact of developing such a tool would be prohibitive.

It remains difficult to determine the exact number of nephrology registered nurses in practice today. A snapshot of the membership profile of the specialty's professional association, the American Nephrology Nurses' Association (ANNA), may provide insight into the areas of practice and positions held by association members. Total membership as of March 31, 2010, was 12,293. The ANNA membership profile is updated annually and available to the members on the ANNA website (www.annanurse.org).

It is difficult to determine the exact number of nephrology nurses in practice today

Areas of Practice

Acute Hemodialysis	5,695	46.3%
Chronic Hemodialysis	8,800	71.6%
Chronic Kidney Disease	3,331	27.1%
Conservative Management	426	3.5%
Cont. Renal Replacement Therapy	1,777	14.5%
Medical-Surgical Unit	1,059	8.6%
Nursing Education	1,618	13.2%
Pediatric Nephrology	733	6.0%
Peritoneal Dialysis	3,550	28.9%
Research	503	4.1%
Therapeutic Apheresis	816	6.6%
Transplantation	1,059	8.6%
Other	1,694	13.8%

Primary Position

Head Nurse/Supervisor	17.7%
Staff/Clinical Nurse	46.7%
Education	7.2%
Administration	8.5%
Clinical Nurse Specialist	2.4%
Coordinator	4.8%
Nurse Practitioner	4.7%
Case Manager	1.5%
Other	6.5%

Since the 1950s, the fast-paced evolution of nephrology care has made continuing education critical to the success of nephrology nurses and the patients they care for

Education and Professional Development

Continuing Education

Registered nurses receive general education on kidney disease in their basic nursing education programs. Additional education for registered nurses interested in nephrology should include content related to acute kidney injury (AKI), patient management, fluid and electrolytes, acid-base balance, pharmacology considerations, and complications. Formal nephrology nursing programs are scarce and limited to specific areas of the country.

The standardization of training continues to be an issue within the specialty. The majority of training and education is delivered at the facility level. The APRN with a specialty in nephrology most often is educationally prepared and certified as a clinical nurse specialist or nurse practitioner. Formal educational programs to prepare APRNs with a specialty in nephrology nursing are limited.

Nephrology registered nurses are accountable for judgments made and actions taken in the course of their nursing practice. Therefore, the process of continuing education is imperative. Since the 1950s, the fast-paced evolution of nephrology care has made continuing education (CE) critical to the success of nephrology nurses and the patients they care for. This process was formally recognized when ANNA was first created and later when nephrology nursing certification was developed. Recertification requirements include attendance or participation in nephrology-specific continuing education programs or activities.

ANNA recognizes the importance of continuing education and offers scholarships that provide funding to support members in their pursuit of higher education.

The National Kidney Foundaton (NFK) hosts the Council of Nephrology Nurses and Technicians (CNNT) that functions as a professional membership council within NFK.

Professional Organization

The American Nephrology Nurses' Association (ANNA) is the specialty's professional association. ANNA was founded over 40 years ago in the late 1960s. Nephrology nurses have consistently supported the endeavors of the organization as it continues to meet their professional needs. The association's mission and values have been updated and revised to reflect the changes in nephrology nursing practice. The current mission and values are noted below.

Mission. ANNA will promote excellence by advancing nephrology nursing practice and positively influence outcomes for individuals with kidney disease.

Values. Integrity • Advocacy • Professional Development • Research

Publications. Additional resources published through the years have enabled ANNA to establish itself as the voice for the nephrology nursing specialty. In 1972, the association published its first *Standards of Clinical Practice,* which addressed hemodialysis, followed in 1974-75 with *Standards of Clinical Practice for Transplantation,* and in 1975-76 with *Standards of Clinical Practice for Peritoneal Dialysis.* Over the years, the standards have been revised to include updated information, structured standards, patient teaching, patient outcomes, and new therapeutic modalities. This edition of ANNA's *Nephrology Nursing Scope and Standards of Practice* incorporates competencies for both the registered nurse and the advanced practice registered nurse working in nephrology.

The *Core Curriculum for Nephrology Nursing* was first published in 1987 and is now in its 5th edition. The textbook, *Contemporary Nephrology Nursing,* was first published in 1998, with its second edition in 2006. In addition to books, the association has published monographs on therapeutic modalities, rehabilitation, and disaster nursing, as well as publications on topics in nephrology nursing research, professional development, and quality assurance.

Position papers developed and published by ANNA have also played an important role in the specialty. Position statements represent succinct summaries of ANNA's stance on a variety of issues for the purpose of influence, advocacy, and/or clarification. Beginning in 1977 with a position paper on the role of the hemodialysis technician, the association has delineated its positions and those of nephrology nursing on a variety of issues including, but not limited to, the scope of practice of nephrology nursing, delegation, certification, and health policy issues. ANNA endorses the recommendations of the National Kidney Foundation Kidney Disease Outcome Quality Initiative (KDOQI) clinical practice guidelines regarding the evaluation, classification, and stratification of CKD.

Certification

In 1986, the ANNA Board of Directors voted to pursue the development of a process to certify proficiency in nephrology nursing practice. With the assistance of the National League of Nursing Testing Service, an ANNA certification ad hoc committee developed a criterion-referenced examination. The exam was designed to ascertain if a nurse who took the exam met the established standard of proficiency in nephrology nursing.

The first test was administered in 1987. In that year, the Certification Ad Hoc Committee evolved to become the Nephrology Nursing Certification Board (NNCB). NNCB was established as a separate corporation with its own bylaws, officers, and board of directors. In 2000, NNCB changed its name to the Nephrology Nursing Certification Commission (NNCC) to reflect a broader scope of certification and recertification activities.

The model of the certification examination for the specialty of nephrology nursing is based on the Dreyfus model of skill acquisition, as adapted by Patricia Benner, to affirm competency in nephrology nursing clinical practice. NNCC bases the development of its examination on practice analyses describing levels of practice and professional development.

ANNA will promote excellence by advancing nephrology nursing practice and positively influence outcomes for individuals with kidney disease

NNCC currrently provides three nephrology nursing certifications:
- CNN – Certified Nephrology Nurse
- CNN-NP – Certified Nephrology Nurse-Nurse Practitioner
- CDN – Certified Dialysis Nurse

Updated requirements are located on the NNCC website (www.nnnc-exam.org).

Health Policy Involvement

Over the years, ANNA has actively participated in the legislative and regulatory arenas. ANNA established its Government Relations Committee in 1981, published its first Legislative Policy Statement in November 1983 (Parker, 1998), developed a state legislative representative program in 1988, and established a legislative office in Washington, D.C., in 1989. Today, ANNA maintains a Health Policy Agenda and a Health Policy Statement, which are reviewed annually.

ANNA developed its Health Policy Committee and a national system of advisors to identify, monitor, and address issues that could affect nursing practice, especially nephrology nursing practice, and/or patients. This system crosses the local, state, and national levels.

In 2003, ANNA held its first End-Stage Renal Disease (ESRD) Education Day. This was a nationwide effort to inform lawmakers about the urgent need to modernize Medicare and help save patients' lives. Lawmakers at the federal, state, and local levels were invited to visit their local dialysis units and learn more about the challenges their constituents face. This education day has evolved into the Kidney Disease Awareness and Education Week (KDAE Week) with increased visits from lawmakers throughout the year.

ANNA hosts the ANNA legislative center where nephrology nurses can quickly identify their legislative representative and communicate electronically on critical issues. ANNA was actively involved in responding to the recent changes in the Medicare and Medicaid programs: the Conditions for Coverage for End-Stage Renal Disease Facilities (CfC) and implementation of the Medicare prospective payment system (PPS) for services to patients with end-stage renal disease.

The current health policy agenda for Medicare ESRD-related issues includes endorsing health policy initiatives that promote organ donation, increase transplantation, prevent chronic kidney disease, and monitor effects of new laws and regulations that impact the ESRD program and its beneficiaries. ANNA also monitors nursing and general health care issues and has responded by supporting increased funding for the Nursing Workforce Development programs and appropriations for the National Institute for Nursing Research (NINR). In addition, ANNA encourages and maintains promotion of safe workplace initiatives, federal and state nursing practice issues and their effects on nephrology nursing, and health care reform proposals.

ANNA continues to support the need to ensure healthcare consumer safety and access to APRNs by aligning education, accreditation, licensure, and certification as shown in the Consensus Model for APRN Regulation: Licensure, Accreditation, Certification, and Education (APRN JDG, 2008). ANNA endorses the specialty certification of the certified nephrology nurse, nurse practitioner (CNN-NP).

Practice Issues

Nephrology nursing practice issues are related to a safe workplace, nursing excellence, and safe practice. It is important to gain a clear understanding of the work environment factors that encourage and discourage the recruitment and retention of qualified nephrology nurses especially in freestanding dialysis units. Evidence from magnet hospital research reveals aspects of the dialysis work environment that may contribute to the shortage of nurses in the hemodialysis unit (Thomas-Hawkins, Flynn, & Clarke, 2008).

Over the years, ANNA has actively participated in the legislative and regulatory arenas

The importance of examining the role of the nephrology nurse is critical in affecting positive patient outcomes and improving the quality and safety of patient care. With this in mind, ANNA funded a study to determine the impact of nephrology registered nurses on patient outcomes.

Findings from that study support the nursing organizations and outcomes model proposition that nephrology RN staffing levels have a significant impact on patient outcomes. The mean patient-to-RN ratio was 9.58 patients per RN: 25% of nurses cared for 4.61 patients or less and 31% of nurses cared for 12 patients or more. Patient-to-RN ratios of 12 or more patients per RN were significantly associated with higher odds of frequent occurrences of shortened and skipped dialysis treatments and patient complaints compared to RNs with the lowest patient-to-RN ratios (i.e., 4.61 or less patients per RN) (Thomas-Hawkins et al., 2008). Two limitations of the study were the wide variation in RN staffing levels and the use of nurse-reported data.

Whether they come from individual corporations or from regulatory agencies, nephrology nurses are constantly faced with the possible implementation of arbitrary staffing ratios. Nephrology nurses need to continue to be diligent in their awareness of pending regulations impacting practice.

Nursing excellence and establishing best practice in all areas of nephrology nursing practice are a focus for the specialty. Interdisciplinary evidence-based guidelines for CKD care are available as a reference to all nephrology practitioners from the National Kidney Foundation Kidney Disease Outcomes Quality Initiative (NFK KDOQI), the Renal Physicians Association (RPA), and the American Nephrology Nurses' Association (ANNA). Nephrology nursing continues to be actively involved as future guidelines are developed.

> **Nephrology nurses regularly evaluate safety, effectiveness, and resources in the planning and delivery of care**

Ethics

Nephrology registered nurses are bound by a professional code of ethics (ANA, 2001) and regulate themselves as individuals through peer review of practice. Nephrology nurses and members of various disciplines in the nephrology community periodically exchange knowledge and ideas about how to deliver high-quality health care, resulting in overlaps and constantly changing professional practice boundaries.

This interdisciplinary team collaboration among health care professionals involves recognition of the expertise of others within and outside one's own profession and referral to those professionals when appropriate. Because of this, nephrology nursing's scope of practice has flexible boundaries.

Nephrology nurses regularly evaluate safety, effectiveness, and resources in the planning and delivery of care. Nephrology nurses recognize that resources are limited and often unequally distributed. Consequently, they try to achieve more equitable distribution and availability of health care services throughout the local community, the country, and the world.

The Centers for Disease Control and Prevention (CDC), the Public Health Department, and ANA are developing crisis standards to be followed during a large-scale disaster. The patient with kidney disease is vulnerable to decreasing health care resources not only in a large-scale disaster, but in the current health care environment constrained by budget shortfalls.

Ethics arise from the necessity of making difficult decisions in the face of conflicting interests. Ethics is now considered an important component of the undergraduate and graduate nursing curriculum. Hospitals are establishing ethics committees to review policies and procedures and provide consultation. All research must be approved by some form of an ethics review board.

Trends and Opportunities

Evidence-Based Practice and Research

Nursing research and evidence-based practice contribute to the body of knowledge and enhances patient outcomes. As a profession, nurses continually evaluate and apply nursing research findings. New knowledge is translated to patient care to promote effective and efficient care and improved patient outcomes. In addition, nurses as a profession ensure practice changes are based on current evidence.

Concurrence with both this publication and the current edition of ANA's *Nursing's Social Policy Statement: The Essence of the Profession* (ANA, 2010c), the nursing profession continually examines nursing practice. An example of this is the study of the freestanding dialysis unit nurse staffing levels, which has demonstrated that safe staffing is imperative to quality patient care. As a specialty practice, we need to continue to determine the work environment factors that encourage or discourage the requirement and retention of qualified nurses in freestanding dialysis units (Thomas-Hawkins, Denno, Currier, & Wick, 2003).

There are opportunities for nephrology nursing in the
- coordination of the transition of the patient to kidney replacement therapies
- education of primary physicians in the timing for referral of the kidney patient to nephrologists and vascular surgeons
- utilization of the APRN in nephrology settings

> Technology offers the promise of creating a better work environment for nurses

Technology

Technology offers the promise of creating a better work environment for nurses when it is designed and implemented in a manner that supports the nurses' work. Ideally, technology eliminates redundancy and duplication of documentation, and reduces probability of errors. The devices used in nephrology nursing are becoming increasingly complex. The nephrology registered nurse needs to have an additional skill set to work not only with specific dialysis equipment but with the new and diverse electronic medical record (EMR) systems. Development of computerized programs that monitor patient outcomes has become commonplace.

Nephrology registered nurses need to be part of the planning and implementation of technology in the workplace. As health care resources become limited, the costs of technology need to be weighed against the benefit to patient care. The nephrology registered nurse needs to be represented when these decisions are made.

Technology can be used in research to improve data collection and analysis as well as to provide information on current patient demographics, comorbidities, and measuring outcomes. Computerized staffing models can provide the nephrology nurse with more time to interact with the patient. The incorporation of any technology, however, is not without risk, and it demands due diligence by nephrology nurses to consider the impact on the scope of nursing practice and the ethical implications for healthcare consumers.

Future of Nephrology Nursing

In the United States, the total number of patients with kidney failure is projected to rise to more than 774,000 patients by 2020 (United States Renal Data System, 2009). Additionally, the current rates of functioning transplants exceed 400 per million in the populations in the United States, Norway, Catalonia, and the Canary Islands. In the United States, there are over 26 million individuals with CKD markers, and millions of others are at risk.

Nephrology registered nurses specializing in the care of patients with kidney disease require a specific body of knowledge as well as complex technical skills. The care that was described in the literature decades ago still serves as the foundation for current care. However, the level of complexity has escalated. The number of patients is increasing. The average age of the patient is rising. The number of comorbidities has dramatically increased.

The impending shortage of nephrology nurses is less of a concern than the loss of the experienced nephrology nurse. The average age of the practicing nephrology nurse continues to increase as does the number of nephrology nurses retiring from the profession. Consequently, the economic and quality of care impacts are considerable. Nephrology nurses have many challenges to face in the future.

A commitment to nephrology nursing requires nurses to remain involved in continuous learning and be accountable for strengthening individual practice through varied practice settings as well as membership in and support of professional associations. The future will show us that

Encroachment of nephrology nursing practice remains a concern

- Nephrology nursing will strengthen the formalized training and education process for the specialty. Formalized education programs in academic nursing programs for advanced practice registered nurses will be available in all areas of the country.
- Nephrology nursing will support the funding of nursing schools to recruit and retain adequate faculty to prepare registered nurses for practice.
- Nephrology nursing will continue to actively encourage nursing research that seeks to examine the specific characteristics of the nephrology work environments, how technology can be used to redesign nephrology workplace environments to meet the needs of patients and the nurses providing their care, and the impact of professional nursing care on patient outcomes.

As we face economic challenges, encroachment of nephrology nursing practice remains a concern. Nephrology nurses underestimate the knowledge they bring to the interdisciplinary team and at times abdicate the leadership role to other disciplines. The future of nephrology nursing depends on the specialty to continue to advocate for the right to lead the interdisciplinary team through continued presence at the "decision-making table."

Nephrology nursing will continue to work independently and as members of coalitions at the state and federal levels to identify and respond to health policy issues that affect the practice of nephrology nurses and the individuals for whom they provide care.

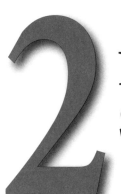

Nephrology Nursing Standards of Practice

Standards

A professional nursing organization has a responsibility to its members and to the public it serves to develop standards of practice. As the professional organization for all nephrology nurses, ANNA has assumed the responsibility for developing standards that apply to the practice of nephrology nurses.

The standards of nephrology nursing practice are authoritative statements of the duties that all nephrology registered nurses are expected to perform competently. The standards contained in this document may serve to gauge the quality of care provided to patients with the understanding that the application of the standards is context dependent. The standards are subject to change with the dynamics of the nursing profession, nephrology practice, and local, state, and federal regulations. In addition, specific conditions and clinical circumstances may affect the application of the standards at a given time (e.g., during a natural disaster). The standards are subject to formal periodic review and revision.

The competencies that accompany each standard may be evidence of compliance with the corresponding standard. The list of competencies is not exhaustive. Whether a particular standard or competency applies depends upon the circumstances. For example, a nephrology nurse providing treatment to a comatose patient with acute kidney injury who has no family present still has a duty to collect comprehensive data pertinent to the patient's health (*Standard 1. Assessment*). However, that nurse would not be expected to assess family composition, history, and dynamics and the impact of those dynamics on the patient's health and wellness (*Standard 1. Assessment Competency*).

Definitions and Concepts Related to Competence (ANA, 2010b)

- An individual who demonstrates competence is performing at an expected level.

- A competency is an expected level of performance that integrates knowledge, skills, abilities, and judgment.

- The integration of knowledge, skills, abilities, and judgment occurs in formal, informal, and reflective learning experiences.

- Knowledge encompasses thinking, understanding of science and humanities, professional standards of practice, and insights gained from context, practical experiences, personal capabilities, and leadership performance.

- Skills include psychomotor, communication, interpersonal, and diagnostic skills.

- Ability is the capacity to act effectively. It requires listening, integrity, knowledge of one's strengths and weaknesses, positive self-regard, emotional intelligence, and openness to feedback.
- Judgment includes critical thinking, problem solving, ethical reasoning, and decision making.

Competence and Competency in Nephrology Nursing Practice

The competent practice of nephrology nursing can be influenced by the nature of the situation, which includes consideration of the setting, resources, and the person. Situations can either enhance or detract from the nephrology registered nurse's ability to perform. The nephrology registered nurse positively influences factors that facilitate and enhance competent practice. Similarly, the nephrology registered nurse seeks to deal with barriers that constrain competent practice. The expected level of performance reflects variability depending upon context and the selected competence framework or model.

The ability to perform at the expected level requires a process of lifelong learning. Nephrology registered nurses must continually reassess their competencies and identify needs for additional knowledge, skills, personal growth, and integrative learning experiences.

STANDARDS OF NEPHROLOGY NURSING PRACTICE

The standards of nephrology nursing practice describe a competent level of nursing care as demonstrated by the application of the nursing process.

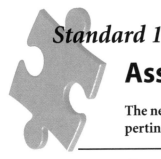

Standard 1

Assessment

The nephrology registered nurse collects comprehensive data pertinent to the healthcare consumer's health and/or the situation.

Competencies

The nephrology registered nurse:

- Provides individualized comprehensive assessment of healthcare consumers and their care needs that contributes to the interdisciplinary team assessment.

- Adheres to applicable federal, state, and local regulations for assessment criteria and frequency for healthcare consumers undergoing kidney replacement therapies (KRTs).

- Collects comprehensive data in a systematic and ongoing process while honoring the uniqueness of the person including, but not limited to, current presentation and health status, including potential risk factors.

Standard 1, continued
Assessment

- Assesses functional level to the extent necessary to determine whether the healthcare consumer is a candidate for referral for further evaluation and possible rehabilitation services.

- Elicits healthcare consumer abilities, interests, values, preferences for modality, setting, self-care, palliative care, expressed needs, knowledge of the health care situation, goals, and expectations for care outcomes.

- Involves the healthcare consumer, family/support system, interdisciplinary team along with other health care providers, and environment, as appropriate, in holistic data collection.

- Identifies barriers (e.g., psychosocial, financial, cultural, language, and educational) to effective communication and makes appropriate adaptations.

- Recognizes impact of personal attitudes, values, and beliefs on care when assessing healthcare consumers with diverse backgrounds or situations.

- Assesses family composition, history, dynamics, and impact on healthcare consumer health and wellness.

- Prioritizes data collection activities based on the healthcare consumer's immediate condition, or anticipated needs of the healthcare consumer or situation.

- Uses appropriate evidence-based assessment techniques, monitors, instruments, and tools in collecting pertinent data.

- Synthesizes available data, information, and knowledge relevant to the situation to identify patterns and variances.

- Applies ethical, legal, and privacy guidelines and policies to the collection, maintenance, use, and dissemination of data and information.

- Recognizes a therapeutic healthcare consumer and provider relationship. Provider honors the healthcare consumer's preferences regarding his or her care.

- Documents relevant data in a retrievable format.

Additional competencies for the advanced practice registered nurse
The advanced practice registered nurse specializing in nephrology:

- Evaluates risks and potential risks of kidney disease in individuals, families, and the community.

- Initiates and interprets diagnostic tests and procedures relevant to the healthcare consumer's current status.

- Assesses the effect of interactions among individuals, family, community, and social systems on health and illness.

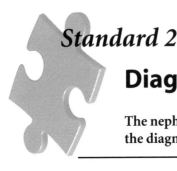

Standard 2

Diagnosis

The nephrology registered nurse analyzes the assessment data to determine the diagnoses or the issues.

Competencies

The nephrology registered nurse:

- Derives the diagnoses or issues based on available assessment data.

- Validates the diagnoses or issues with the healthcare consumer, family, and interdisciplinary team when possible and appropriate or during comprehensive care planning development.

- Identifies actual or potential risks to the healthcare consumer's health and safety or barriers to health that may include, but are not limited to, interpersonal, systematic, or environmental circumstances.

- Uses standardized classification systems and clinical decision support tools, when available, in identifying diagnoses.

- Focuses on healthcare consumer response to kidney replacement therapy, prevention, or slowing progression of kidney disease, renal complications, comorbidities, and/or palliative care.

- Documents diagnoses or issues in a manner that facilitates the determination of the expected outcomes and the plan that meets requirements of dialysis-related licensing and regulatory agencies.

Additional competencies for the advanced practice registered nurse

The advanced practice registered nurse specializing in nephrology:

- Systematically compares and contrasts clinical findings with normal and abnormal variations and developmental events in formulating a differential diagnosis and intervenes when appropriate.

- Utilizes complex data and information obtained during interview, examination, and diagnostic procedures in identifying diagnoses.

- Uses the CKD staging classification system to document specific CKD diagnosis.

- Assists staff in developing and maintaining competence in the diagnostic process.

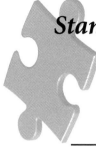

Standard 3

Outcomes Identification

The nephrology registered nurse identifies expected outcomes for a plan individualized to the healthcare consumer or the situation.

Competencies

The nephrology registered nurse:

- Involves the healthcare consumer, family, interdisciplinary team along with other health care providers in formulating expected outcomes when possible and appropriate.

- Derives ethnic and culturally appropriate expected outcomes from the diagnoses.

- Considers associated risks, benefits, costs, current scientific evidence, expected trajectory of the condition, and clinical expertise when formulating expected outcomes.

- Develops outcomes consistent with current scientific evidence-based practice, clinical practice standards, and applicable regulatory guidelines.

- Uses evidence-based tools during review of records for a ready reference of the current professionally accepted clinical practice standards to establish targets for individual clinical outcomes for healthcare consumers undergoing kidney replacement therapy (KRT).

- Defines expected outcomes in terms of the individual healthcare consumer, the healthcare consumer's culture, values, ethical considerations, environment, and/or situation in relationship to the associated risks, benefits, cost, and scientific evidence.

- Includes a time estimate for attainment of expected outcomes.

- Develops expected outcomes that facilitate continuity of care.

- Modifies expected outcomes based on changes in the status of the healthcare consumer or evaluation of the situation.

- Documents expected outcomes as measurable goals.

Additional competencies for the advanced practice registered nurse

The advanced practice registered nurse specializing in nephrology:

- Identifies expected outcomes that incorporate scientific evidence and are achievable through implementation of evidence-based practices.

- Identifies expected outcomes that incorporate cost and clinical effectiveness, healthcare consumer satisfaction, and continuity and consistency among providers.

- Supports the use of clinical guidelines and evidence-based practices linked to effective individual healthcare consumer outcomes.

- Differentiates outcomes that require care process interventions from those that require system-level interventions.

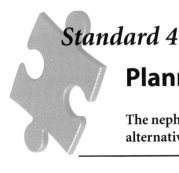

Standard 4

Planning

The nephrology registered nurse develops a plan that prescribes strategies and alternatives to attain expected outcomes.

Competencies

The nephrology registered nurse:

- Develops an individualized plan in partnership with the interdisciplinary team that establishes goals and priorities for care while considering healthcare consumer characteristics (e.g., stage of CKD, vascular access type, acuity, transplant status, and/or other unique healthcare consumer needs).

- Incorporates an implementation pathway or timeline within the plan.

- Establishes the plan priorities with the healthcare consumer, family, the interdisciplinary team, and others, as appropriate.

- Includes strategies in the plan that address each of the identified diagnoses or issues. These strategies may include strategies for:
  - Promotion and restoration of health
  - Prevention of illness, injury, and disease
  - Alleviation of suffering
  - Supportive care for those who are dying

- Includes strategies for health and wholeness across the lifespan.

- Provides for continuity in the plan.

- Considers the economic impact of the plan on the healthcare consumer, family, caregivers, or other affected parties.

- Integrates current scientific evidence, trends, and research.

- Utilizes the plan to provide direction to other members of the health care team.

- Explores practice settings, staffing resources, and safe space and time to explore suggested, potential, and alternative options.

- Defines the plan to reflect best practices, statutes, rules and regulations, and standards.

- Modifies the plan according to the ongoing assessment of the healthcare consumer's response and other outcome indicators.

- Documents the plan in a manner that uses standardized language or recognized terminology.

Additional competencies for the advanced practice registered nurse

The advanced practice registered nurse specializing in nephrology:

- Identifies barriers to care, assessment strategies, diagnostic strategies, and therapeutic interventions within the plan that reflect current evidence, including data, research, literature, and expert clinical knowledge.

Standard 4, continued
Planning

- Selects or designs strategies to meet the multifaceted needs of complex healthcare consumers.

- Includes the synthesis of the healthcare consumer's priorities, values, and beliefs regarding nursing and medical therapies within the plan.

- Leads the design and development of interdisciplinary processes to address the identified diagnosis or issue.

- Actively participates in the development and continuous improvement of systems that support the planning process.

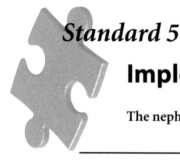

Standard 5

Implementation

The nephrology registered nurse implements the identified plan.

Competencies

The nephrology registered nurse:

- Partners with the healthcare consumer, family, significant others, interdisciplinary team, and others to implement and integrate the plan in a safe, realistic, timely manner.

- Demonstrates caring behaviors toward healthcare consumers, significant others, and groups of people receiving care.

- Utilizes technology to measure, record, and retrieve healthcare consumer data, implement the nursing process, and enhance nephrology nursing practice.

- Documents implementation and any modification, including changes or omissions, of the identified plan.

- Utilizes evidence-based interventions and treatments specific to the diagnosis or problem.

- Provides holistic care according to the stage of kidney disease while addressing the needs of the diverse healthcare consumer across the lifespan.

- Advocates for health care that is sensitive to the needs of healthcare consumers, with particular emphasis on the needs of diverse populations.

- Applies appropriate knowledge of major health problems and cultural diversity in implementing the plan of care.

- Applies available health care technologies to maximize access and optimize outcomes for healthcare consumers.

- Utilizes community resources and systems to implement the plan.

- Collaborates with health care providers from diverse backgrounds to implement and integrate the plan.

- Accommodates for different styles of communication used by healthcare consumers, families, and health care providers.

Standard 5, continued
Implementation

- Integrates traditional and complementary health care practices as appropriate.

- Implements the plan in a timely manner in accordance with patient safety goals.

- Promotes the healthcare consumer's capacity for the optimal level of participation and problem solving.

- Documents implementation and any modifications, including changes or omissions, of the identified plan.

Additional competencies for the advanced practice registered nurse
The advanced practice registered nurse specializing in nephrology:

- Facilitates utilization of systems, organizations, and community resources to implement the plan.

- Supports collaboration with nursing and other colleagues to implement the plan.

- Incorporates multiple ways of knowing (empirical, personal, ethical, socio-political and aesthetic) and strategies to initiate change in nursing care practices if desired outcomes are not achieved.

- Assumes responsibility for the safe and efficient implementation of the plan.

- Uses advanced communication skills to promote relationships between nurses and healthcare consumers, to provide a context for open discussion of the healthcare consumer's experiences, and to improve the healthcare consumer's outcomes.

- Actively participates in the development and continuous improvement of systems that support the implementation of the plan.

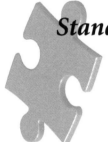

Standard 5a

Coordination of Care

The nephrology registered nurse coordinates care delivery.

Competencies
The nephrology registered nurse:

- Organizes the components and coordinates the implementation of the plan.

- Manages care to meet the special needs of healthcare consumers with kidney disease to maximize independence and quality of life.

- Assists the healthcare consumer to identify options for alternative care.

- Communicates the plan with other health care providers, the healthcare consumer, family, and system through written documentation and verbal communication, as necessary, during transitions in care.

- Advocates for the delivery of dignified and humane care by the interdisciplinary team.

- Documents the coordination of care.

Standard 5a, continued
Coordination of Care

Additional competencies for the advanced practice registered nurse
The advanced practice registered nurse specializing in nephrology:

• Provides leadership in the coordination of interdisciplinary health care for integrated delivery of healthcare consumer care services.

• Synthesizes data and information to prescribe necessary system and community support measures, including modifications of surroundings.

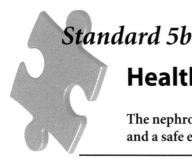

Standard 5b

Health Teaching and Health Promotion

The nephrology registered nurse employs strategies to promote health and a safe environment.

Competencies

The nephrology registered nurse:

• Provides health teaching that addresses such topics as healthy life styles, risk-reducing behaviors, devleopmental needs, activities of daily living, and preventive self-care.

• Uses health promotion and health teaching methods appropriate to the situation, stage of CKD, treatment modality, the healthcare consumer's developmental level, learning needs, readiness, ability to learn, language preference, spirituality, culture, and socioeconomic status.

• Seeks opportunities for feedback and evaluation of the effectiveness of the strategies used.

• Uses information technologies to communicate health promotion and disease prevention information to the healthcare consumer in a variety of settings.

• Provides healthcare consumers with information about intended effects and potential adverse effects of proposed therapies.

• Collaborates in the design and provides early chronic kidney disease education in advance of kidney replacement therapy (KRT) that includes information on all modalities including self-care dialysis and transplantation.

• Educates healthcare consumers with kidney disease and their families on kidney replacement options, palliative care, and rationale for the medical management plan.

• Provides education on kidney disease to the public, people at risk for kidney disease, and other community groups.

Additional competencies for the advanced practice registered nurse
The advanced practice registered nurse specializing in nephrology:

• Synthesizes empirical risk behaviors, learning theories, behavioral change theories, motivational theories, epidemiology, and other related theories and frameworks when designing health education information and programs.

• Conducts personalized health teaching and counseling considering comparative effectiveness research recommendations.

Standard 5b, continued
Health Teaching
and Health Promotion

- Designs health information and healthcare consumer education appropriate to the healthcare consumer's development level, learning needs, readiness to learn, and cultural values and beliefs.

- Evaluates health information resources, such as the Internet, within the area of practice for accuracy, readability, and comprehensibility to help healthcare consumers access quality health information.

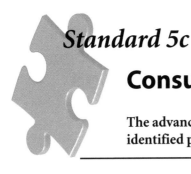

Standard 5c

Consultation

The advanced practice registered nurse provides consultation to influence the identified plan, enhance the abilities of others, and effect change.

Competencies

The advanced practice registered nurse specializing in nephrology:

- Synthesizes clinical data, theoretical frameworks, and evidence when providing consultation.

- Facilitates the effectiveness of a consultation by involving the healthcare consumer and other stakeholders in decision making and negotiating role responsibilities.

- Communicates consultation recommendations.

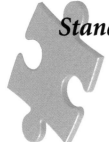

Standard 5d

Prescriptive Authority and Treatment

The advanced practice registered nurse uses prescriptive authority, procedures, referrals, treatments, and therapies in accordance with state and federal laws and regulations.

Competencies

The advanced practice registered nurse specializing in nephrology:

- Prescribes evidence-based treatments, therapies, and procedures, considering the healthcare consumer's comprehensive health care needs.

- Prescribes pharmacologic agents based on state practice acts and current knowledge of pharmacology and physiology.

- Prescribes specific pharmacologic agents and/or treatments based on clinical indicators, the healthcare consumer's status and needs, known contraindications including allergies, and when appropriate, the results of diagnostic and laboratory tests.

Standard 5d, continued
Prescriptive Authority and Treatment

- Prescribes pharmacologic agents taking into account the effects of abnormal kidney function and drug metabolite accumulation.

- Evaluates therapeutic and potential adverse effects of pharmacologic and nonpharmacologic treatments.

- Provides healthcare consumers with information about intended effects and potential adverse effects of proposed prescriptive therapies.

- Provides information about costs and alternative treatments and procedures, as appropriate.

- Evaluates and incorporates complementary and alternative therapy into education and practice.

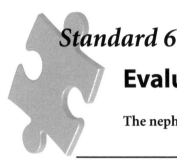

Standard 6

Evaluation

The nephrology registered nurse evaluates progress toward attainment of outcomes.

Competencies

The nephrology registered nurse:

- Conducts a systematic, ongoing, and criterion-based evaluation of the outcomes in relation to the structures and processes prescribed by the plan and the indicated timeline.

- Collaborates with the individual healthcare consumer and others involved in the care or situation in the evaluative process.

- Evaluates, in partnership with the individual healthcare consumer, the effectiveness of the planned strategies in relation to healthcare consumer responses and the attainment of the expected outcomes.

- Uses ongoing assessment data to revise the diagnoses, outcomes, the plan, and implementation, as needed.

- Disseminates results to the healthcare consumer, family, and others involved in the care or situation, as appropriate, in accordance with state and federal laws and regulations.

- Participates in assessing and assuring the responsible and appropriate use of interventions, equipment, and monitors to minimize unwarranted or unwanted treatment and healthcare consumer suffering.

- Reevaluates the appropriateness of the current modality ability for self-care, referral to vocational and physical rehabilitation services, and all other criteria mandated by the CMS Conditions for Coverage and Interpretive Guidelines for healthcare consumers undergoing KRT.

- Documents the results of the evaluation.

Additional competencies for the advanced practice registered nurse
The advanced practice registered nurse specializing in nephrology:

- Evaluates the accuracy of the diagnosis and effectiveness of the interventions in relationship to the healthcare consumer's attainment of expected outcomes.

- Synthesizes the results of the evaluation analyses to determine the effect of the plan on healthcare consumers, families, groups, communities, institutions, networks, and organizations.

- Adapts the plan of care for the trajectory of treatment based on evaluation of response.

- Uses the results of the evaluation analyses to make or recommend process or structural changes, including policy, procedure, or protocol documentation and revision, as appropriate.

STANDARDS OF PROFESSIONAL PERFORMANCE

The Standards of Professional Performance describe a competent level of behavior in the professional role, including activities such as enhancement of quality of practice, continuing education, professional practice evaluation, collaboration, integration of ethics, research, resource utilization, and leadership. All registered nurses are expected to engage in professional role activities, including leadership, appropriate to their education, experience, and position. Nephrology registered nurses are accountable for their professional actions to themselves, their healthcare consumers, their peers, and ultimately, to society.

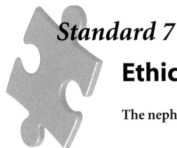

Standard 7

Ethics

The nephrology registered nurse practices ethically.

Competencies

The nephrology registered nurse:

• Uses the *Guide to the Code of Ethics for Nurses: Interpretation and Application* (ANA, 2010a) to guide practice.

• Delivers care in a manner that preserves and protects healthcare consumer autonomy, dignity, rights, values, and beliefs.

• Recognizes the centrality of the healthcare consumer and family as core members of any health care team.

• Upholds and advocates for healthcare consumer confidentiality within legal and regulatory parameters.

• Assists healthcare consumers in self determination and informed decision making.

• Maintains therapeutic and professional healthcare consumer–nurse relationship with appropriate professional role boundaries.

• Takes appropriate action regarding instances of illegal, unethical, or inappropriate behavior that can endanger or jeopardize the best interests of the healthcare consumer or situation.

• Speaks up when appropriate to question health care practice when necessary for safety and quality improvement.

• Recognizes that nephrology professionals have frequent encounters with ethical dilemmas due to the nature of the specialty (appropriateness of kidney replacement therapy including initiation, withdrawal/withholding of treatment, decisional capacity, preexisting advance directives, and resource allocation).

Standard 7, continued
Ethics

- Advocates for equitable healthcare consumer care.

- Contributes to resolving ethical issues/moral distress of healthcare consumers, colleagues, or systems, as evidenced in such activities as participating on ethics committees, comprehensive healthcare consumer care conference, and Quality Assessment and Performance Improvement (QAPI) meetings.

Additional competencies for the advanced practice registered nurse
The advanced practice registered nurse specializing in nephrology:

- Practices with interdisciplinary teams that address ethical risks, benefits, and outcomes.

- Provides information on the risks, benefits, and outcomes of health care regimens to allow informed decision making by the healthcare consumer, including informed consent and informed refusal.

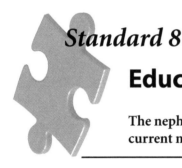

Standard 8

Education

The nephrology registered nurse attains knowledge and competence that reflects current nursing practice.

Competencies
The nephrology registered nurse:

- Participates in ongoing educational activities related to appropriate knowledge bases and professional issues.

- Demonstrates a commitment to lifelong learning through self-reflection and inquiry to address learning and personal growth needs.

- Seeks experiences that reflect current practice to maintain knowledge, skills, abilities, and judgment in clinical practice or role performance.

- Acquires knowledge and skills appropriate to the nephrology role, practice setting, or situation.

- Seeks formal and independent learning experiences to develop and maintain professional skills and knowledge.

- Identifies learning needs based on nursing knowledge, the various roles the nurse may assume, and the changing needs of the healthcare consumer with kidney disease.

- Participates in formal or informal consultations to address issues in nephrology nursing practice as an application of education and knowledge base.

- Shares educational findings, experiences, and ideas with peers.

- Contributes to a work environment conducive to the education of health care professionals.

- Maintains professional records that provide evidence of competency and lifelong learning.

Standard 8, continued
Education

Additional competencies for the advanced practice registered nurse
The advanced practice registered nurse specializing in nephrology:

- Uses current health care research findings and other evidence to expand clinical knowledge, skills, abilities, and judgment to enhance role performance, and increase knowledge of professional issues.

- Provides education and serves as a resource to educate nurses and other groups on the subject of kidney disease management.

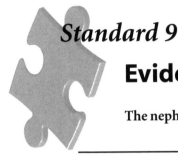

Standard 9

Evidence-Based Practice and Research

The nephrology registered nurse integrates evidence and research findings into practice.

Competencies
The nephrology registered nurse:

- Utilizes current evidence-based nursing knowledge, including research findings, to guide practice.

- Incorporates evidence when initiating changes in nursing practice.

- Participates, as appropriate to education level and position, in the formulation of evidence-based practice through research.

- Shares personal or current evidence-based research findings from reputable sources with colleagues and peers.

Additional competencies for the advanced practice registered nurse
The advanced practice registered nurse specializing in nephrology:

- Contributes to nursing knowledge by conducting or synthesizing research and other evidence that discovers, examines, and evaluates current practice, knowledge, theories, criteria, and creative approaches to improve health care practice.

- Promotes a climate of research and clinical inquiry.

- Disseminates research findings through activities, such as presentations, publications, consultation, and journal clubs.

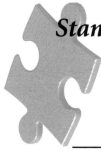

Standard 10

Quality of Practice

The nephrology registered nurse contributes to quality nursing practice.

Competencies

The nephrology registered nurse:

- Demonstrates quality by documenting the application of the nursing process in a responsible, accountable, and ethical manner.

- Uses creativity and innovation in nephrology nursing practice to improve care delivery.

- Participates in quality improvement activities. Such activities may include:

  - Identifying aspects of practice important for quality monitoring (e.g., early and ongoing healthcare consumer education regarding vascular access care).

  - Using indicators developed to monitor quality and effectiveness of nursing practice (e.g., intradialytic and posttreatment hypotensive episodes).

  - Collecting data to monitor quality and effectiveness of nephrology nursing practice.

  - Analyzing quality data to identify opportunities for improving nursing practice and care of the healthcare consumer with kidney disease.

  - Formulating evidence-based recommendations to improve nephrology nursing practice or outcomes.

  - Implementing activities to enhance the quality of nephrology nursing practice.

  - Developing, implementing, and/or evaluating policies, procedures, and/or guidelines to improve the quality of nephrology nursing practice.

  - Participating on and/or leading interdisciplinary teams to evaluate clinical care or health services for healthcare consumers with kidney disease.

  - Participating in and/or leading efforts to minimize costs and unnecessary duplication of services.

  - Identifying problems that occur in day-to-day work routines to correct process inefficiencies.*

  - Analyzing factors related to safety, satisfaction, effectiveness, and cost/benefit options.

  - Analyzing organizational systems for barriers to quality healthcare consumer outcomes.

- Implementing processes to remove or decrease barriers within organizational systems.
- Participates in professional association activities.

Additional competencies for the advanced practice registered nurse
The advanced practice registered nurse specializing in nephrology:

- Provides leadership in the design, implementation, and monitoring of quality improvement activities.

Standard 10, continued
Quality of Practice

- Designs innovations to effect change in nephrology nursing practice and improve health outcomes.

- Evaluates the practice environment and quality of nursing care rendered in relation to existing evidence.

- Identifies opportunities for the generation and use of research and evidence.

- Obtains and maintains professional certification.

- Uses the results of quality improvement activities to initiate changes in nephrology nursing practice and in the health care delivery system.

* Board of Higher Education & Massachusetts Organization of Nurse Executives, 2006

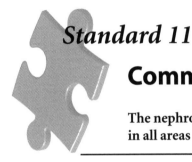

Standard 11

Communication

The nephrology registered nurse communicates effectively in a variety of formats in all areas of practice.

Competencies

The nephrology registered nurse:

- Assesses communication format preferences of healthcare consumers, families, and colleagues.*

- Assesses her or his own communication skills in encounters with healthcare consumers, families, and colleagues.*

- Seeks continuous improvement of her or his own communication and conflict resolution skills.*

- Conveys information to healthcare consumers, families, the interdisciplinary team, and others in communication formats that promote accuracy.

- Questions the rationale supporting care processes and decisions when they do not appear to be in the best interest of the patient.*

- Discloses observations or concerns related to hazards and errors in care or the practice environment to the appropriate level.

- Maintains communication with other providers to minimize risks associated with transfers and transition in care delivery.

- Contributes her or his own professional perspective in discussions with the interdisciplinary team.

* Board of Higher Education & Massachusetts Organization of Nurse Executives, 2006

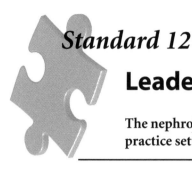

Standard 12

Leadership

The nephrology registered nurse demonstrates leadership in the professional practice setting and the profession.

Competencies

The nephrology registered nurse:

- Oversees the care given by others while retaining accountability for the quality of care given to the healthcare consumer.

- Abides by the vision, the associated goals, and the plan to implement and measure progress of an individual healthcare consumer or progress within the context of the health care organization.

- Demonstrates a commitment to continuous, lifelong learning education for self and others.

- Mentors colleagues for the advancement of nephrology nursing practice, the nursing profession, and quality health care.

- Treats colleagues with respect, trust, and dignity.*

- Develops communication and conflict resolution skills.

- Participates in key roles on committees, councils, and administrative teams.

- Participates in professional organizations.

- Seeks ways to advance nursing's autonomy and accountability.*

- Communicates effectively with healthcare consumers and colleagues.

- Participates in efforts to influence health care policy on behalf of consumers and the profession.

- Develops and implements a succession plan to ensure continuity of care.

Additional competencies for the advanced practice registered nurse
The advanced practice registered nurse specializing in nephrology:

- Influences decision-making bodies to improve the nephrology nursing practice environment and healthcare consumer outcomes.

- Provides direction to enhance the effectiveness of the interdisciplinary team.

- Promotes advanced practice nursing in nephrology and role development by interpreting its role for healthcare consumers, families, and others.

- Models expert practice to nurses, other interdisciplinary team members, and healthcare consumers.

- Mentors colleagues in the acquisition of clinical knowledge, skills, abilities, and judgment.

- Participates in designing systems that support effective teamwork and positive outcomes.

* Board of Higher Education & Massachusetts Organization of Nurse Executives, 2006

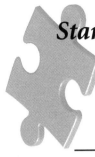

Standard 13

Collaboration

The nephrology registered nurse collaborates with the healthcare consumer, family, and others in the conduct of nephrology nursing practice.

Competencies

The nephrology registered nurse:

- Partners with others to effect change and generate positive outcomes through the sharing of knowledge of the healthcare consumer and/or situation.
- Communicates with healthcare consumers, family, and health care providers regarding healthcare consumer care and the nurse's role in the provision of that care.
- Promotes conflict management and resolution.
- Participates in building consensus or resolving conflict in the context of patient care.
- Applies group process and negotiation techniques with healthcare consumers and colleagues.
- Adheres to standards and applicable codes of conduct that govern behavior among peers and colleagues to create a work environment promoting cooperation, respect, and trust.
- Cooperates in creating a documented plan focused on outcomes and decisions related to care and delivery of services that indicate communication with healthcare consumers, families, and others.
- Engages in teamwork and team-building processes.

Additional competencies for the advanced practice registered nurse

The advanced practice registered nurse specializing in nephrology:

- Partners with other disciplines to enhance healthcare consumer outcomes through interdisciplinary activities, such as education, consultation, management, technological development, or research opportunities.
- Invites the contribution of the healthcare consumer, family, and team members to achieve optimal outcomes.
- Leads in establishing, improving, and sustaining collaborative relationships to achieve safe, quality health care for the consumer.
- Documents plan of care communications, rationales for plan of care changes, and collaborative discussions to improve healthcare consumer outcomes.

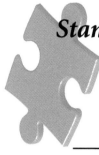

Standard 14

Professional Practice Evaluation

The nephrology registered nurse evaluates her or his own nursing practice in relation to professional practice standards and guidelines, relevant statutes, rules, and regulations.

Competencies

The nephrology registered nurse:

- Provides age-appropriate and developmentally appropriate care in a culturally and ethnically sensitive manner.

- Engages in self-evaluation of practice on a regular basis, identifying areas of strength as well as areas in which professional growth would be beneficial.

- Obtains informal feedback regarding one's own practice from healthcare consumers, peers, professional colleagues, and others.

- Participates in peer review, as appropriate.

- Takes action to achieve goals identified during evaluation process.

- Provides the evidence for practice decisions and actions as part of the informal and formal evaluation processes.

- Interacts with peers and colleagues to enhance one's own professional practice or role performance.

- Provides peers with formal or informal constructive feedback regarding their practice or role performance.

Additional competencies for the advanced practice registered nurse

The advanced practice registered nurse specializing in nephrology:

- Engages in a formal processes seeking feedback regarding her or his own practice from healthcare consumers, peers, professional colleagues, and others.

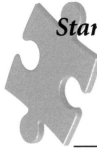

Standard 15

Resource Utilization

The nephrology registered nurse utilizes appropriate resources to plan and provide nursing services that are safe, effective, and financially responsible.

Competencies

The nephrology registered nurse:

- Assesses individual healthcare consumer care needs and resources available to achieve desired outcomes.

- Identifies healthcare consumer care needs, potential for harm, complexity of the task, and desired outcome when considering resource allocation.

- Delegates elements of care to appropriate health care workers in accordance with any applicable legal policy parameters or principles.

- Identifies the evidence when evaluating resources.

- Advocates for resources, including technology, that enhance nephrology nursing practice.

- Modifies practice when necessary to promote a positive interface among healthcare consumers, care providers, and technology.

- Assists the healthcare consumer and family in identifying and securing appropriate and available services to address needs across the health care continuum.

- Assists the healthcare consumer and family in factoring costs, risks, and benefits in decisions around treatment and care.

Additional competencies for the advanced practice registered nurse

The advanced practice registered nurse specializing in nephrology:

- Utilizes organizational and community resources to formulate interdisciplinary plans of care.

- Formulates innovative solutions for healthcare consumer care problems that utilize resources effectively and maintain quality.

- Designs evaluation strategies to demonstrate cost effectiveness, cost benefit, and efficiency factors associated with nephrology nursing practice.

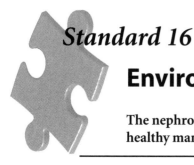

Standard 16

Environmental Health

The nephrology registered nurse practices in an environmentally safe and healthy manner.

Competencies

The nephrology registered nurse:

- Attains knowledge of environmental health concepts, such as implementation of environmental health strategies.
- Promotes a practice environment that reduces environmental health risks of workers, healthcare consumers, and the general public.
- Assesses the practice environment for factors such as air quality, sounds, odor, noise obstacles, temperature, and light that negatively affect the healthcare consumer.
- Advocates for the judicious and appropriate use of products used in delivery of health care.
- Advocates for appropriate staffing patterns that will provide safe, quality care and reduce staff burnout.
- Communicates environmental health risks and exposure reduction strategies to the healthcare consumers, families, colleagues, and communities.
- Utilizes scientific evidence to determine if a product or treatment is a potential environmental threat.
- Participates in strategies to promote healthy communities.
- Takes actions to prevent/report a hostile work environment.
- Immediately seeks help to resolve potentially volatile situations.
- Promotes and monitors the practice environment for appropriate infection control practices including consumer safety, environmental, and equipment concerns, which impact the healthcare consumer.

Additional competencies for the advanced practice registered nurse

The advanced practice registered nurse specializing in nephrology:

- Creates partnerships that promote sustainable environmental health policies and conditions.
- Analyzes the impact of social, political, and economic influences upon the environment and human health exposures.
- Critically evaluates the manner in which environmental health issues are presented by the popular media.
- Advocates for implementation of environmental principles for nursing practice.
- Supports nurses in advocating for and implementing environmental principles in nephrology nursing practice.

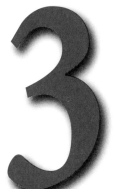

3 How to Use the Standards in Practice

The *Nephrology Nursing Scope and Standards of Practice* delineates the professional responsibilities of nephrology nurses engaged in nursing practice regardless of the setting. As such, it can serve as a basis for

- Quality improvement systems
- Regulatory systems
- Health care reimbursement and financing methodologies
- Development and evaluation of nursing service delivery systems and organizational structures
- Certification activities
- Position descriptions and performance appraisals
- Agency policies, procedures, and protocols
- Educational offering goals and objectives
- Establishing the legal standard of care

It is imperative to continue to examine how nephrology standards of professional nursing practice can be disseminated and used more effectively to enhance and promote the quality of nephrology nursing practice. In addition, standards of nephrology nursing practice must be evaluated on an ongoing basis and revised as necessary to reflect current best practices and technology changes. The dynamic nature of the health care practice environment and the growing body of nursing research provide both the impetus and the opportunity for nephrology nursing to ensure competent nephrology nursing practice in all settings and to promote ongoing professional development that enhances the quality of nephrology nursing practice.

This section provides the nephrology nurse with examples of how to incorporate the *Nephrology Nursing Scope and Standards of Practice* into clinical practice. There is no limit to its application. These are some examples of situations where referencing the standards enhances nephrology nursing practice.

The following forms are examples and should be modified to meet individual needs of the facility. Please go to **www.annanurse.org/StandardsForms** to download these documents for personal use. The documents are password protected. Enter the password **NephrologyNurse** when prompted.

Disclaimer

These forms were created for educational purposes only. They are intended to provide examples of the types of forms that administrators and nephrology registered nurses may want to use to incorporate the *Nephrology Nursing Scope and Standards of Practice* into clinical practice. The information provided is not intended to establish or replace forms provided by dialysis providers to their facilities. Please check with your manager before implementing any form provided here.

It is the responsibility of the user to verify that the use of any of the forms does not violate copyright laws.

Performance Appraisal Action Plan

A nurse manager can use the *Nephrology Nursing Scope and Standards of Practice* when providing an employee with corrective action. Based on *Standard 1. Assessment*, an appropriate assessment is the collecton of comprehensive data pertinent to the healthcare consumer's health and/or the situation. If the nephrology nurse does not document the data, the standard is not met.

Using the *Nephrology Nursing Scope and Standards of Practice*, the manager can review the competencies for *Standard 1. Assessment*. The manager can then document the specific competency in which the nurse is deficient. The standard and related competencies can be used to develop the action plan for correction of the deficiency.

No Name Dialysis Center

Performance Appraisal Action Plan

Employee Name: _____   Title: _____

Manager's Name: _____   Location/Department: _____

The purpose of this action plan is to identify the behavior(s), performance dimension, or skill(s) that must be improved or developed to meet position expectations. The following strategies outline opportunities for improvement or development. The expectation is that the manager and employee meet periodically (biweekly, monthly) to review progress on action plan components and make necessary changes or revisions as needed.

Dimension Identify area, skill, rated as needs improvement on evaluation	Action Include recommendations	Timeframe/Completion Deadline
Mary will document the following when completing patient assessments. (Use facility policy.) Assessment of the Dialysis Patient • The nephrology registered nurse collects comprehensive data pertinent to the healthcare consumer's health and/or the situation. (Standard 1. Assessment)	• Synthesizes available data, information, and knowledge relevant to the situation to identify patterns and variances. • Documents relevant data in a retrievable format.	• Completes on 100% of primary care patients over the next 90 days.
2.		
3.		
4.		

Employee Signature: _____   Date: _____

Manager Signature: _____   Date: _____

Individual Development Plan (IDP)

Facilities or individual nephrology nurses interested in promoting professional development can apply the standards to the development of an Individual Development Plan (IDP). The IDP can be formulated annually and discussed at an annual review. The *Nephrology Nursing Scope and Standards of Practice* provide an important tool for the nephrology nurse interested in developing short- and long-term career objectives.

Using *Standard 8. Education* and *Standard 12. Leadership* can assist with the completion of the nurse's IDP. When *Standard 8. Education* is reviewed, the nurse finds two goals that can be completed within a shorter time frame, and describes the activities that will be completed and a method of application of the knowledge gained. *Standard 12. Leadership* is used to begin the process of developing leadership skills. The following IDP tool reflects the nurse's goals:

- Over the next 1 to 2 years, the nurse has a goal of maintaining her or his certification status by attending continuing educational offerings.
- The nurse has a longer term goal of developing leadership competencies and supporting her local ANNA chapter in a leadership role.

No Name Dialysis Center				
Individual Development Plan (IDP)				
Section 1				
Name:			Date:	
Title & Location:			Employee ID:	
Section 2 – Short-range Goals (1–2 years)				
Goal	**Developmental Activity/Training**	**How Will Knowledge Be Applied**	**Completion Date**	**Status**
These goals are taken directly from the competencies section of the Standards for Professional Performance: ***Standard 8: Education.*** 1. Participates in ongoing educational activities related to appropriate knowledge bases and professional issues. 2. Seeks experiences that reflect current practice to maintain knowledge, skills, abilities, and judgment in clinical practice or role performance.	1. Will attend two ANNA-sponsored conferences within the calendar year. 2. Volunteer to actively participate on No Name Dialysis Center's Quality Improvement Committee.	1. Will present to fellow nephrology nurses information obtained at the conferences. 2. Will assist in improving clinical practice skills.		1. Initiated 2. Active participant
Section 3 – Long-range Career Goals (2–5+ years)				
Goal	**Developmental Activity/Training**	**How Will Knowledge Be Applied**	**Completion Date**	**Status**
This goal was taken directly from the competencies section of the Standards for Professional Performance: ***Standard 12: Leadership.*** 1. Mentors colleagues for the advancement of nephrology nursing practice, the nursing profession, and quality health care.	1. Volunteer at the local ANNA Chapter assisting developing educational conferences for ANNA members.	1. Assists in developing leadership skills which may be used to mentor colleagues in nephrology nursing.		1. Not initiated at this time
Section 4				
Signature:			Date:	
Supervisor Signature:			Date:	

Employee Performance Review Form

A local area administrator is having a difficult time designing a performance review for the nursing staff. Recalling that the *Nephrology Nursing Scope and Standards of Practice* address Standards of Professional Performance, the administrator decides to use these to evaluate the nursing staff.

The administrator collaborates with the facility staff, and they decide that ethics, leadership, communication, collaboration, quality practice, and environmental health are the areas they will use to evaluate nursing care. Each standard indicates competencies and these will be incorporated into the performance review form. In addition, the administrator added several key components that were mandated to be included by the corporate office.

No Name Dialysis Center
Employee Performance Review Form

Employee Name	Job Title	Job Date / /	Review Period / / thru / /

Rating System

TT = Top Talent: Performance exceeds position requirements. Results attained, values clearly demonstrated, and personal contribution is exceptional.

VC = Valued Contributor: Performance meets position requirements. Results attained and personal contribution represent the level expected.

NI = Needs Improvement: Performance requires improvement in order to meet position requirements. ACTION PLAN REQUIRED.

Position-Specific Requirements

Review job description to determine overall rating for job-specific requirements including essential functions, technical competencies, and job-specific knowledge.

Rate results attained for job-specific objectives (**attach applicable job description**):

Ethics *From Standard 7 Ethics* The nephrology registered nurse practices ethically. Please note, (E) = employee's self-evaluation rating, and (M) = manager's rating.	Rating E M	*Communication/Collaboration* *From Standard 11 Communication; Standard 13 Collaboration* The nephrology registered nurse communicates effectively in a variety of formats in all areas of practice. And collaborates with healthcare consumer, family and others in the conduct of nursing practice. Please note, (E) = employee's self-evaluation rating, and (M) = manager's rating.	Rating E M
Uses the *Guide to the Code of Ethics for Nurses: Interpretation and Application* (ANA, 2010) to guide practice.		Partners with others to effect change and generate positive outcomes through the sharing of knowledge of the healthcare consumer and/or situation.	
Delivers care in a manner that preserves and protects healthcare consumer autonomy, dignity, rights, values, and beliefs.		Adheres to standards and applicable codes of conduct that govern behavior among peers and colleagues to create a work environment promoting cooperation and respect.	
Assists healthcare consumers in self determination and informed decision making.		Maintains communication with other providers to minimize risks associated with transfers and transition of care delivery.	
Maintains therapeutic and professional healthcare consumer-nurse relationship with appropriate professional role boundaries.		Uses scripts for key customer encounters.	
Safe Environment *From Standard 16 Environmental Health* The nephrology registered nurse practices in an environmentally safe and healthy manner.	Rating E M	Follows up on customer requests and issues.	
Takes action to prevent/report a hostile work environment.		Looks for opportunities to increase customer satisfaction with service.	
Promotes and monitors the practice environment for appropriate infection control practices including consumer safety, which impact the healthcare consumer.		Greets coworkers, visitors and patients with a smile and "Hello."	
Maintains adherence to dress code.		Answers every call with a greeting – "Good Morning/Afternoon" and states facility and name.	
		Closes each interaction by asking, "Is there anything else I can do for you?"	
Maintains a safe environment in relation to patient age and physical condition.			

Continues on next page

Employee Performance Review Form, continued

Quality of Practice From Standard 10 The nephrology registered nurse contributes to quality nursing practice. Please note: (E) = employee's self-evaluation rating and (M) = manager's rating	Rating E	M	Leadership From Standard 12 The registered nephrology nurse demonstrates leadership in the professional practice setting and the profession. Please note: (E) = employee's self-evaluation rating and (M) = manager's rating	Rating E	M
Demonstrates quality by documenting the application of the nursing process in a responsible, accountable, and ethical manner.			Oversees the nursing care given by others while retaining accountability for the quality of care given to the healthcare consumer.		
Uses creativity and innovation in nephrology nursing practice to enhance nursing care.			Treats others with respect, trust, and dignity.		
			Develops positive working relationships with coworkers.		
			Displays reliability and punctuality.		
			Shares ideas and contributes time to help others (internal and external) of department.		

Performance Highlights/Comments Use this section to record individual pertinent information from the review and comments regarding achievements, accomplishments, strengths, changes in duties, and development areas. Please note, (E) = employee's self-evaluation rating, and (M) = manager's rating	Rating E	M

Job-Specific Objectives: Use this section to record individual goals for the upcoming year that are job-specific. They can be related to change in responsibilities, developing new skills, improving a particular skill, projects, assignments, etc.	

No Name Dialysis Center Employee Requirements

Department Competencies Met	( ) yes	( ) no
Age-Specific Competencies Met (if applicable)	( ) yes	( ) no
PPD Requirement Met	( ) yes	( ) no
Safety Day Requirement Met	( ) yes	( ) no
Fit Test Requirement Met (if applicable)	( ) yes	( ) no
Attendance Requirement Met	( ) yes	( ) no
HIPAA Confidentiality Requirement Met	( ) yes	( ) no
Dress Code Requirement Met	( ) yes	( ) no
Corporate Compliance Awareness Met	( ) yes	( ) no

Values Grid (use colors)

Blue is Exceeds Standard/Role Model; **Green** is Consistently Meets Standard; **Red** is Does not Meet Standard/Needs Improvement

Integrity	Respect	Caring	Excellence	Commitment	Teamwork

Examples of Blue Values and Red Values in Practice
Caring – Always takes the time to speak with patients and educate families (this is blue) Commitment – Often calls out leaving the staff short of Registered Nurses on weekends (this is red)

Continues on next page

Employee Performance Review Form, continued

Behaviors that this individual should KEEP doing:	
Behaviors this individual should STOP doing:	
Behaviors this individual should START doing:	
The next career step(s) for this individual is(are):	

Performance Discussion & Planning

Current Rating	
Top Talent	☐
Valued Contributor	☐
Needs Improvement	☐

My personal contribution to No Name Dialysis Center's mission for the coming year is:

1.

2.

Employee's Signature	Date	Supervisor's Signature	Date

For ratings of Top Talent and Needs Improvement, signature of next level manager is required:

Next Level Signature _____   Date _____

Policy and Procedure Development

The No Name Dialysis Center has had several episodes with disputes between staff members and patients. On several occasions, the No Name Dialysis Center's administrator had to intervene to provide conflict resolution to resolve patient issues. The No Name Dialysis Center recognizes the need to develop a policy to resolve issues and disputes that arise within the dialysis unit. After reviewing the Standards of Practice, *Standard 16: Environmental Health,* the following competencies are noted:

- Participates in strategies to promote healthy communities.
- Takes actions to prevent/report a hostile work environment.
- Immediately seeks help to resolve potentially volatile situations.

Based upon this standard, the following policy was created. While the policy is lengthy, it includes the Standard of Professional Performance to be expected within the dialysis facility.

No Name Dialysis Center			
Policy and Procedure			
MANUAL TITLE(S)		Page __ of ___	**Attachments**
MANUAL SECTION	**MANUAL SUBJECT**		
DATE OF ISSUE	**DATE OF REVISION(S)**	**EFFECTIVE DATE**	

PURPOSE: Violence Prevention Program

POLICY

- The safety and security of personnel, patients, and visitors is of vital importance. Therefore, acts or threats of physical violence, including intimidation, harassment, or coercion, which occurs on No Name Dialysis Center property will not be tolerated.

- This prohibition against threats and acts of violence applies to all persons involved, including, but not limited to, employees, supervisors, physicians, students, contract and temporary personnel, patients, and visitors. Therefore, violations of this policy by any individual on No Name Dialysis Center property are considered misconduct and will lead to disciplinary and/or legal action as appropriate.

- No reprisals will be taken against any employee who reports or experiences workplace violence.

- All No Name Dialysis Center personnel must refrain from engaging in acts of violence and are responsible for maintaining a work environment free from acts or threats of violence.

- Violence Prevention Program Elements:

  - **Conducting an annual assessment** of No Name Dialysis Center property which includes facility layout, access control, and lighting; crime in the surrounding community; communication equipment; emergency response capabilities

  - **Controlling access to facilities and sensitive areas**

  - **Ensuring adequate security systems** including card readers, cameras, door locks, windows, physical barriers, and restraint systems are operational and appropriate for the setting

  - **Maintaining effective systems to warn others** of a security danger or to summon assistance (i.e., panic buttons)

  - **Providing adequately trained staff** to provide services and response

  - **Conducting an Annual Security Opinion Survey** to obtain feedback on services and identify opportunities for improvement

  - **Reviewing all incidents** involving security-assisted restraints, disorderly persons, thefts, and assaults. Action plans are developed, implemented, and monitored as appropriate

  - **Enforcing Visitor Control** and identification policies

  - **Providing Preventing Workplace Violence and Nonviolent Crisis Intervention**/Identification and Management of Aggressive Behavior courses through No Name Dialysis Center corporate office

* *The above bolded areas reflect elements of* Standard 16. Environmental Health.

Continues on next page

Policy and Procedure – Violence Prevention Program, continued

Response to Potential Violence

- **When a threat of violence is identified,** a team will be formed to review information and determine the appropriate actions. The team will consist of members from the following departments:
  Human Resources
  Nursing
  Security Department
  Risk Management/Legal
  Public Relations
  Social Work/Behavioral Health
  Administration
  Purchasing

- The team's duties include, but are not limited to:
  - **Reviewing past incidents** of aggression or violence and identifying the threat level
  - **Referring to the Warning Sign** and Appropriate Response to Aggressive Behavior for guidance
  - **Reviewing the facility's readiness** to respond to issues of aggression or violence
  - **Ensuring adequate security** presence and response is available
  - **Establishing liaison** with local law enforcement and emergency services
  - **Communicating to employees** or others that were or may be involved in an incident involving workplace violence
  - **Assigning all or some** of these tasks to other individuals

- **Managers and supervisors** are responsible for the following:
  - Providing workplace violence prevention training for personnel under their supervision
  - Assisting management response team as necessary

- **Reporting Requirements**
  - Employees/Supervisors
  Personnel shall immediately report any acts or threats of violence to the Security Department, their supervisor/manager, or to the Human Resources Department. Employees are additionally required to report the occurrences of each warning sign of violence that they observe (i.e., verbal abuse, aggressive behavior, loitering). No employee will be disciplined or discharged for reporting any threats or acts of violence.

- **Contracted Services**
  - Third parties working on No Name Dialysis Center property shall be informed of Workplace Violence Prevention requirements by purchasing prior to doing any actual work on hospital premises.

- **Postincident Management**
  - Victims of violence will receive immediate physical evaluations, be removed from the worksite, and treated for acute injuries. Additionally, referrals shall be made for appropriate evaluation, treatment, counseling, and assistance both at the time of the incident and for any follow-up treatment necessary.

- **Record Keeping**
  - Record keeping should be used to provide information for analysis, evaluation of methods of control, severity determinations, identifying training needs, and overall program evaluations. Record keeping includes the following:
    - ✔ **Entry of injury on the OSHA Injury and Illness Log.** Injuries that must be recorded include the following:
      - Loss of consciousness
      - Restriction of work or motions
      - Transfer to another job or termination of employment
      - Medical treatment beyond first aid

Continues on next page

Policy and Procedure – Violence Prevention Program, continued

✔ **All incidents of abuse, verbal attacks, or aggressive behavior**

✔ **Recording and communicating mechanism** so that staff who provide care for an escalating or potentially aggressive, abusive, or violent patient will be aware of the patient's status and of any problems experienced in the past

✔ **Gathering of information** to identify any past history of violent behavior, incarceration, probation reports, or any other information that assists employees to assess violent status

✔ **Training program** contents and sign-in sheets of all attendees are maintained

Warning Signs and the Appropriate Response to Aggressive Behavior
The following is a guideline for determining the severity of a violent situation and the appropriate response.

Procedure

LOW
These are behaviors that should raise the awareness of the employees and others around the employee, patient, or visitor. It is an indication that a problem is developing and will likely continue without intervention.

Behavioral Examples
> Inappropriate behavior
> Abusive language
> Excessive use of profanity
> Argumentative
> Lack of cooperation when requests are made
> Sexual comments, gestures, or innuendoes
> Negative attitude toward the rules
> Frequent displays of anger
> Emotionally erratic
> Veiled threats
> Inappropriate use of computers and phone systems

Recommendations
- *Employee*
  Document incident and notify supervisor
  Supervisor and Human Resources reviews behavioral expectations with employee
  Consult with Human Resources if behavior continues
  Coach/counsel employee

- *Patient*
  Document incident
  Notify supervisor and security
  Discuss with physician and social worker

- *Visitor*
  Document incident
  Notify supervisor
  Notify security
  Consider visitor restriction or supervised visits

Continues on next page

Policy and Procedure – Violence Prevention Program, continued

MEDIUM

These are behaviors that should sound the alarm that the situation is escalating and that without intervention, an incident could occur.

Behavioral Examples

Overt, covert, or indirect threats
Expressed desire to do harm to others
Attempts to instigate fights
Open defiance of the rules
Vandalism
Property theft
Belief that others are conspiring against them or prosecuting them
Sexual or violent notes sent to others
Expressed suicidal thoughts or threats
Physical acting out of anger
Comments about weapons or stories of harming others
Severe emotional distress

Recommendations

- *Employee*
  Obtain assistance and guidance from Human Resources, Legal, and Behavioral Health Leadership
  Document all incidents and assist in the investigation
  Coach/counsel employee

- *Patient*
  Document incident
  Notify supervisor and security
  Discuss appropriate intervention with physician, nurse, and social worker

- *Visitor*
  Document incident
  Notify supervisor and security
  Notify local law enforcement and consult Legal

HIGH

These are behaviors that are dangerous and require immediate intervention and assistance.

Behavioral Examples

Clear intent to harm
Physical assault
Intense uncontrollable anger
Overt threats to kill
Showing a weapon
Sabotage with intent to harm others
Suicide attempt

Recommendations

- *Employee*
  Call the local police (911) and security and notify Human Resources for guidance
  Ensure the safety of all employees, patients, and visitors
  Document the incident and assist in the investigation

Continues on next page

Policy and Procedure – Violence Prevention Program, continued

- *Patient*
  Assign 1:1
  Expedite medical treatment
  Contact network

- *Visitor*
  Document incident
  Notify supervisor and security
  Notify legal and local police department

EXTREME
This is a situation where there is on-going or imminent danger due to physical or armed aggression. Employee should seek safety, call police (911), and stay calm.

Physician order required:	No
Consent required:	No
Who may perform:	RNs, technicians, and other dialysis facility personnel
Who may assist:	RNs, technicians, and other dialysis facility personnel
Current Evidence:	Participates in strategies to promote healthy communities. * Takes actions to prevent/report a hostile work environment. * Immediately seeks help to resolve potentially volatile situations. * * *Standard 16. Environmental Health*
Equipment/Supplies:	Not required
Age-specific technical consideration:	Age-specific considerations should be taken into account when type and level of Aggressive Behavior is evaluated.
Documentation:	As noted under each level response to *Warning Signs and the Appropriate Response to Aggressive Behavior*

APPROVED BY:	DATE APPROVED:
SOURCE:	CONCURRED:
DISTRIBUTION: See Distribution list	KEYWORDS:

Position Description

The nursing staff of the No Name Dialysis Center was asked to develop a position description for the registered nurse. The charge nurse had a copy of the *Nephrology Nursing Scope and Standards of Practice*, which they used as a reference. The nursing staff was able to create a position description that included many of the standards within the role statement and job essentials. The role statement includes assessment, diagnosis, plan, implementation, and evaluation of patient care.

The nursing staff also added outcomes identification, ethics, education, and evidence-based practice. The nurse manager was impressed with the development of the position description and that the nurses included the *Nephrology Nursing Scope and Standards of Practice* within their position description.

No Name Dialysis Center
Job Description

Position Title: Registered Nurse

Reports to: Nurse Manager   **Department**: Nursing

Role Statement *
Responsible for assessing, diagnosing, planning, implementing, and evaluating patient care through outcome identification and evidence-based practice. As an integral member of the health care team, coordinates patient care and communicates and collaborates extensively with the other members of the health care team, patients and/or patient's family or significant other(s). Maintains and demonstrates high standards of professional ethics.
* Incorporates Standards 1, 3, 4, 5, 6, 7, 9, 13

Job Essentials *
• Performs an assessment of the patient, leading to development, implementation, and evaluation of a plan of care
• Administers, monitors, and documents therapeutic interventions and regimens
• Effectively manages rapidly changing situations
• Participates in clinical decision-making
• Educates patient and family/responsible party regarding disease process, individual care needs, wellness, safety issues, etc.
• Delegates and monitors care rendered by other members of nursing department and health care team
• Demonstrates standard precautions and patient safety principles in practice
• Participates in orientation, education, and development of health care team
• Identifies and participates in performance improvement activities
• Maintains professional and departmental level competencies
* Incorporates Standards 1, 3, 4, 5, 8, 10, 11, 13, 14, 16

Educational Requirements, Qualifications
• Graduate of an accredited school of nursing
• Valid RN license in the state of practice (refer to the educational/regulatory requirement of each state)
• Demonstrates knowledge of nursing skills, facility/hospital practices, procedures, and standards
• Assessment skills, ongoing education
• Strong communication skills
• Coordinate and collaborate with a team of health care providers

Job Description
Americans with Disabilities Act (ADA) Requirements:
(Based on a Scale of I to V, with V being the highest level)
• Physical Strength – IV
• Manual Dexterity – IV
• Motor Coordination – III
• Form Perception – IV
• Environmental Conditions – I
   – Environmental hazards – Potential exposure to toxic or caustic chemicals, infectious diseases, radiant energy, electric shock, proximity to moving, mechanical parts, and exposure to combative behavior.
   – Physical demands – Talking and hearing, vision, stooping, kneeling, crouching, reaching, handling, feeling, fingering.
   – Machines, equipment, work aids which may be representative, but not all-inclusive of those commonly associated with this type of work – electric beds, cardiac monitors, stretchers, wheel chairs, sharp objects, i.e., needles and syringes, oxygen and suction equipment, and other medical equipment, computers, and other office equipment.

Competency Skills Checklist

The mentor of the No Name Transplant Center was asked by the Department Supervisor to develop a skills checklist. The mentor used the *Nephrology Nursing Scope and Standards of Practice* in the development of the skills checklist. He identified the outcomes for transplant nurses based on the standards of assessment and planning.

Competency Skills Checklist

Form Guidelines

Purpose:
Use this form to outline one or more competencies. List only critical performance criteria to evaluate.

1. Print all demographic information as listed.

2. Place a check mark in the box indicating the age requirement(s) related to this competency based on the population served by the department.

3. State the title of the competency to be evaluated under Performance Criteria.

4. State the selected Performance Criteria in behavioral terminology in the performance criteria column.

5. Enter the validation method(s) selecting from the alphabetical key on the form.

6. Enter "ME" for Meets Expectations or "NI" for Needs Improvement in the Evaluation column.

7. Use the Comment Line to indicate follow-up plan if evaluation indicates need for improvement.

8. The validator signs and dates the form in the space provided.

Attach and send form to Human Resources with Performance Appraisal

No Name Transplant Center

Job/Population Specific Competency Skills Checklist (Clinical)

Name/Title _____ Dept/Unit _____

Employee ID Number _____ Division _____ Date: _____/_____/_____

Ages: Neonate (< 30 days) Preschool (3-5 years) Adulthood (18-69 years)
Infant (1 month to 1 year) School age (6-12 years) Later Adult (>70 years)
Toddler (1-3 years) Adolescent (13-18 years)

Validation Method: A = Policy Review F = Case Study Exam K = N/A
B = Direct Observation G = Documentation Review
C = Video Review H = Self Learning Module (SLP)
D = Verbalization I = Simulated Demonstration
E = Written Exam J = Other (specify)

Performance Criteria	Validation Method (May use more than one method)	Evaluation		Comments
Assessment of Renal Transplant Recipient		**Meets Expectations**	**Needs Improvement**	
Identifies barriers (such as psychosocial, financial, cultural, language, and educational) to effective communication and makes appropriate adaptations. (*Standard 1. Assessment*)	B. Documents findings in nursing assessment form within 12 hrs of admission			
Provides for and promotes continuity in the plan. (*Standard 4. Planning*)	F. Prepares and revises nursing care plan that reflects assessment findings			
Prioritizes data collection activities based on the healthcare consumer's immediate condition, or anticipated needs of the healthcare consumer or situation. (*Standard 1. Assessment*)	A. Follows No Name Transplant Center P&P on patient identification and completion of surgical checklist			
Synthesizes available data, information, and knowledge relevant to the situation to identify patterns and variances. (*Standard 1. Assessment*)				
Uses appropriate evidenced-based assessment techniques, instruments, and tools. (*Standard 1. Assessment*)				

Employee Signature: _____ Date: _____/_____/_____

Validator Signature: _____ Date: _____/_____/_____

Send to HR with Performance Appraisal

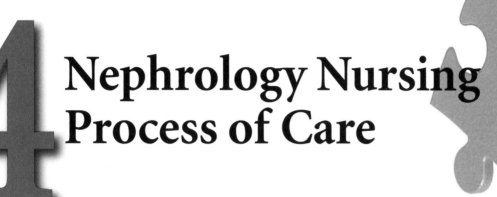

Nephrology Nursing Process of Care

Guidelines are systematically developed statements that have a potential for improving the quality of clinical and healthcare consumer decision making. They are based on available scientific evidence, clinical expertise, and expert opinion. Guidelines address specific patient populations or phenomena where standards have a broader framework for practice.

The question to ask: "Is nephrology nursing ready to develop guidelines today?" The answer: "No, not yet." To be credible, guidelines need to conform to established research criteria and provide documentation of the quality and quantity of evidence. The National Guideline Clearinghouse is an established source of guidelines. Tools are available to guide organizations in the development of guidelines. The tools include the Appraisal of Guidelines and Research and Evaluation (AGREE) and the Conference on Guideline Standardization (COGS) checklist (Newhouse, 2010).

We are not the only specialty in need of improvement in the quality of guidelines. Currently, most of the guidelines are largely based on expert opinion instead of research evidence. Therefore, in this publication we have outlined the nursing process for care of the patient with kidney disease. These processes are based on recommendations from the updated National Kidney Foundation Kidney Disease Outcome Quality Initiative (KDOQI), Kidney Disease: Improving Global Outcomes (KDIGO), the Renal Physician Association (RPA), and ANNA clinical practice guidelines on kidney replacement and end-of-life care as well as opinions of nephrology nursing experts.

Nephrology Nursing Processes of Care

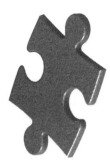

Chronic Kidney Disease, Stages 1–4

CKD is a progressive loss in kidney function over a period of months or years.

Stages of chronic kidney disease

Stage Description	GFR Level
Normal kidney function	Healthy kidneys 90 mL/min or more
Stage 1	Kidney damage with normal or high GFR 90 mL/min or more
Stage 2	Kidney damage and mild decrease in GFR 60 to 89 mL/min
Stage 3	Moderate decrease in GFR 30 to 59 mL/min
Stage 4	Severe decrease in GFR 15 to 29 mL/min
Stage 5	Kidney failure less than 15 mL/min or on dialysis

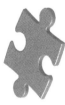

Anemia

Patient Outcomes

The patient will achieve and maintain hemoglobin (Hb) and hematocrit (Hct) within the targeted ranges.

The patient will demonstrate a reduction in modifiable risk factors for development of cardiovascular disease (CVD).

The patient will demonstrate knowledge concerning anemia in chronic kidney disease (CKD): its treatment, risk associated with anemia, and with the treatment of anemia.

Nursing Care

Assessment

1. Assess the patient's
   A. Weight at each health encounter
   B. Blood pressure (BP) and heart rate at each health encounter
   C. Respiratory rate and quality
   D. Skin and mucous membranes
   E. Ability to follow medication regimen

Anemia

2. Assess the patient for signs or symptoms of anemia
   A. Angina, hypotension, tachycardia, shortness of breath
   B. Decreased energy and activity levels
   C. Diminished appetite and weight loss
   D. Lessened sense of well-being
   E. Diminished sexual interest and function
3. Review laboratory test results
   A. Blood urea nitrogen (BUN) and creatinine, and estimated glomerular filtration rate (eGFR)
   B. Complete blood count (CBC) including red blood cell indices (mean corpuscular hemoglobin [MCH], mean corpuscular volume [MCV], mean corpuscular hemoglobin concentration [MCHC]), white blood cell count (WBC), differential and platelet count
   C. Iron profile (i.e., iron, ferritin, total iron binding capacity [TIBC], iron, transferrin saturation [TSAT], and reticulocyte hemoglobin content [CHr]saturation)
   D. Albumin
   E. Folate and B_{12} levels
4. Assess patient for potential causes of anemia
   A. Blood loss
   B. Iron deficiency
   C. Vitamin deficiencies
   D. Inflammation or infection
   E. Secondary hyperparathyroidism
   F. Malnutrition
   G. Medications
   H. Existing medical conditions
   I. Hospitalization
5. Assess patient's understanding of anemia

Collaborate with health care professionals to develop and use an anemia management protocol for CKD

Intervention

1. Collaborate with health care professionals including nephrologist and advanced practice nurse to develop and use an anemia management protocol for CKD
2. Ensure medications are administered as prescribed including iron supplements, vitamins, and erythropoeisis-stimulating agents (ESA)
3. Monitor response to therapy including Hb, Hct, and iron profile. Frequency of monitoring is based on therapy response and goals
4. Monitor blood pressure, particularly during initiation of erythropoietin therapy and report elevations to physician or advanced practice nurse
5. Encourage adherence to medication regimen
6. Identify resources to assist patient to achieve goals of anemia management
7. Request or initiate consultations or referrals as appropriate

Patient Teaching

Before teaching begins, consider health literacy and individualize the approach by considering patient's cultural and health beliefs, preferences, and wishes

1. Educate patient regarding
   A. Kidney function and its relationship to anemia
   B. Signs and symptoms of anemia
   C. Consequences of anemia, including left ventricular hypertrophy (LVH)
   D. Diagnostic tests used to evaluate anemia

Anemia

E. Signs of bleeding
   (1) hematemesis
   (2) tarry stool
F. Iron and vitamin levels and their effects on erythropoiesis
G. Management of anemia of CKD, including iron administration and erythropoietin therapy

Advanced Practice Nursing Care

(In addition to items outlined above)

Assessment

1. Estimate the patient's GFR using a prediction equation at each health encounter if appropriate
2. Interpret results of obtained diagnostic studies (e.g., laboratory tests, electrocardiogram [EKG], echocardiogram)
3. Initiate an anemia assessment in accordance to KDOQI guidelines or facility protocol
4. Monitor patient's ability to follow the treatment plan
5. Maintain Hb in target range as per anemia management protocol
6. Monitor patient's response to treatment plan
7. Monitor patient for causes of hyporesponse
   A. Infection and inflammation
   B. Blood loss
   C. Secondary hyperparthyrodism
   D. Vitamin deficiency
   E. Malnutrition
   F. Medication interactions
8. Monitor patient's BP
9. If anemia related to cancer, collaborate with oncologist

Treat anemia of CKD considering most recent KDOQI clinical practice guidelines

Intervention

1. Treat anemia of CKD considering most recent KDOQI clinical practice guidelines
   A. Establish target Hb (National Kidney Foundation, 2007a))
   B. Initiate an anemia workup
   C. Develop and use an anemia management protocol
2. Evaluate patient for comorbid conditions such as angina, pulmonary disease, hypotension, congestive heart failure, or cerebrovascular disease, and collaborate with physician to establish higher target Hb if appropriate
3. Order laboratory tests and diagnostic studies as appropriate
4. Adjust medication regimen based on patient response
5. Adjust BP medications as indicated for increased BP
6. Consult hematology if cause of hyporesponse is not evident

References

National Kidney Foundation. (2000a). K/DOQI clinical practice guidelines for anemia of chronic kidney disease: Update 2000. *American Journal of Kidney Diseases, 37*(1)(Suppl. 1), S182-S238. Erratum in: (2001). *American Journal of Kidney Diseases, 38*(2), 442.

National Kidney Foundation. (2006a). KDOQI clinical practice guidelines and clinical practice recommendations for anemia of chronic kidney disease. *American Journal of Kidney Diseases, 47*(5)(Suppl. 3), S1-S145.

National Kidney Foundation. (2007a). KDOQI clinical practice guidelines for anemia of chronic kidney disease: 2007 update of hemoglobin target. *American Journal of Kidney Diseases, 50*(3), 471-530.

Chronic Kidney Disease – Mineral and Bone Disorder (CKD-MBD)

Patient Outcomes

The patient will maintain mineral biochemical parameters and acid-base balance within the targeted range.

The patient will be free of disability related to bone disease, calcific cardiovascular abnormalities, and other soft tissue calcification.

The patient will demonstrate knowledge of CKD-MBD and its complications including bone disease, calcific cardiovascular abnormalities, and soft tissue calcification.

The patient will demonstrate knowledge of his or her role in prevention, management, and progression of CKD-MBD.

Nursing Care

Assessment

1. Assess the patient's
   A. Muscle strength, gait, and range of motion, noting limitations in movement
   B. Height or linear growth (pediatric patient)
   C. Joints for enlargement, swelling, stiffness, and tenderness
   D. Bone pain
   E. Skin for local tissue injury or presence of macules, papules, or pruritis
   F. Eyes for visible irritation and local inflammation
   G. Extremities for presence and quality of pulse and vascular insufficiency
   H. Blood pressure and heart rate
   I. Adherence to diet and medication regimens
2. Assess the patient for
   A. Risk factors for osteoporosis
      (1) advancing age
      (2) postmenopausal status
      (3) race
      (4) nutritional vitamin D deficiency
      (5) medications
      (6) malignancy
      (7) prolonged immobilization
   B. History of injuries, the progression of healing, and the potential for new injuries
   C. Financial constraints in meeting dietary and medication regimens
3. Assess the patient's environment for potential hazards
4. Review laboratory obtained test results for
   A. Serum calcium
   B. Phosphorus
   C. Calcium-phosphorus product
   D. Alkaline phosphatase
   E. CO_2
   F. 25-OH vitamin D

CKD-MBD

G. Parathyroid hormone (PTH)

H. Aluminum level

5. Review results of diagnostic tests
    A. Bone x-rays and dual energy x-ray absorptiometry (DEXA) in patients with fractures or known risk factors for osteoporosis
    B. Discuss x-ray results in patient with signs of vascular calcification with health care provider (HCP)
    C. Discuss electrocardiogram (EKG) and echocardiogram results with HCP

6. Assess patient's understanding of bone and mineral disorder

Intervention

1. Collaborate with nephrologist, advanced practice nurse, dietitian, and primary care provider in planning appropriate dietary and medication regimens
2. Restrict dietary phosphorus if phosphorus levels are elevated
3. Ensure medications are administered as prescribed including phosphate binder, calcium supplement, and alkali salts
4. Administer vitamin D according to prescribed treatment plan and monitor for hypercalcemia and oversuppression of PTH
5. Encourage adherence to prescribed dietary and medication regimens
6. Collaborate with social worker regarding financial assistance as needed for dietary and medication regimens
7. Collaborate with physical therapy for aids for mobility as appropriate
8. Identify resources to assist patient to achieve bone metabolism goals
9. Ensure patient's home environment has been evaluated for safety issues (falls)
10. Request or initiate consultations and referrals as appropriate

Encourage adherence to prescribed dietary and medication regimens

Patient Teaching

Before teaching begins, consider health literacy and individualize the approach by considering patient's cultural and health beliefs, preferences, and wishes

1. Educate patient regarding
    A. Kidney function and its relationship to disorders of bone metabolism
    B. Consequences of alterations in bone metabolism
        (1) CKD bone disease
        (2) extraskeletal calcification
        (3) development of cardiovascular disease
    C. Signs and symptoms of
        (1) disorders of bone metabolism
        (2) extraskeletal calcification
        (3) hypo- and hyperphosphatemia
        (4) hypo- and hypercalcemia
    D. Timing of medications related to meals
    E. Reductions of mobility hazards in the home and work environment
    F. Exercise to maintain strength and mobility
    G. Prevention and management of CKD bone disease and extraskeletal calcification

Advanced Practice Nursing Care

(In addition to items outlined above)

Assessment

1. Estimate the patient's GFR using a prediction equation at each health encounter
2. Interpret results of diagnostic studies

3. Monitor patient's ability to follow the treatment plan
4. Monitor patient's response to treatment plan (diet modifications, phosphate binders, calcium supplements, vitamin D supplements, and alkali salts)
5. Monitor for development of CKD bone disorder and signs of extraskeletal calcification

Intervention

1. Treat disorders of CKD-MBD following the KDOQI clinical practice guidelines (2003 or most recent updates) and the KDIGO clinical practice guidelines (2009 or most recent update)
   A. Dietary modifications and prescription
   B. Prescribe and monitor medications
   C. Monitor development of CKD bone disorder and extraskeletal calcification
2. Order diagnostic studies and frequency of testing as appropriate (e.g., laboratory tests, x-ray, DEXA [stages 1-2], EKG, echocardiogram)
3. Adjust medication regimen as appropriate, based on biochemical parameters and patient response
4. Adjust diet prescription based on patient assessment findings

References

Kidney Disease: Improving Global Outcomes. (2009). Clinical practice guidelines for the diagnosis, evaluation, prevention, and treatment of chronic kidney disease-mineral and bone disorder (CKD-MBD). *Kidney International, 76*(Suppl. 113), S1-130.

National Kidney Foundation. (2003a). K/DOQI clinical practice guidelines for bone metabolism and disease in chronic kidney disease. *American Journal of Kidney Diseases, 42*(4)(Suppl. 3), S1-S201.

Uhlig, K., Berns, J., Kestenbaum, B., Kumar, R., Leonard, M., Martin, K., Sprague, S., & Goldfarb, S. (2009). US commentary on the 2009 KDIGO clinical practice guideline for diagnosis, evaluation, and treatment of CKD-mineral and bone disorder (CKD-MBD). *American Journal of Kidney Disease, 55*(5), 773-799.

Dyslipidemia and Reduction of Cardiovascular Disease Risk Factors

Patient Outcomes

The patient will achieve and maintain lipoprotein levels within the targeted ranges.

The patient will demonstrate a reduction in modifiable risk factors for development of cardiovascular disease (CVD).

The patient will demonstrate knowledge of dyslipidemia and cardiovascular risk factor reduction.

Nursing Care

Assessment

1. Assess the patient's
   A. Weight at each health encounter
   B. Body mass index (BMI) initially and then, at a minimum, annually
   C. Blood pressure and heart rate
   D. Apical and peripheral pulses
   E. Respiratory rate and quality

Dyslipidemia – Cardiovascular

    F. Peripheral edema

    G. Lifestyle habits, including smoking, alcohol consumption, and exercise frequency

    H. Adherence to dietary and medication regimens

2. Assess the patient for major CVD risk factors
    A. Cigarette smoking
    B. Hypertension
    C. Low high-density lipoprotein (HDL) (<40mg/dL or 0.40 g/L)
    D. Family history of premature coronary heart disease (CHD)
        (1) CHD in father or brother <55 years old
        (2) CHD in mother or sister <65 years old
    E. Age
        (1) men >45 years old
        (2) women >55 years old
    F. History of myocardial infarction (MI), arrhythmia
    G. Hormone replacement therapy (HRT)
3. Assess patient for CVD risk factors in CKD
    A. Anemia
    B. Hyperhomocysteinemia
    C. Disorders of bone metabolism
    D. Volume overload
4. Review laboratory values
    A. Blood urea nitrogen (BUN) and creatinine
    B. Total cholesterol, low density lipoprotein (LDL), high density lipoprotein (HDL)
    C. Triglycerides
    D. Hemoglobin and hematocrit
    E. Calcium, phosphorous, and parathyroid hormone (PTH)
    F. Homocysteine level
5. Assess patient's understanding of dyslipidemia and reduction of cardiovascular disease risk factors

Identify resources to assist patient to achieve goals of lipid management

Intervention

1. Collaborate with nephrologist, advanced practice nurse, dietitian, and primary care provider in identifying patients at risk for CVD and in planning risk factor reduction, therapeutic lifestyle changes (TLC), dietary, and medication regimens
2. Ensure medications are administered as prescribed, including aspirin, vitamins, and lipid-lowering drugs
3. Encourage adherence to TLC
4. Encourage adherence to diet, fluid restriction, and medication regimen
5. Identify resources to assist patient to achieve goals of lipid management
6. Request or initiate consultations and referrals as appropriate

Patient Teaching

Before teaching begins, consider health literacy and individualize the approach by considering patient's cultural and health beliefs, preferences, and wishes

1. Educate patient regarding
    A. Kidney function and its relationship to lipoprotein levels
    B. Lipoprotein levels and their effect on preservation of kidney function and development of CVD
    C. Modifiable risk factors for CVD and risk reduction
        (1) cessation of smoking
        (2) control of hypertension

Dyslipidemia – Cardiovascular

      (3) control of bone metabolism
      (4) fluid control
      (5) treatment of anemia

D. Therapeutic lifestyle changes (TLC) – involve patient family/support system in teaching regarding diet and exercise
      (1) diet and weight management
      (2) increased physical activity
      (3) moderation in alcohol consumption

Advanced Practice Nursing Care

(In addition to items outlined above)

Assessment

1. Estimate the patient's GFR using a prediction equation at each health encounter
2. Assess the patient for CHD risk-equivalent conditions
    A. Clinical CHD
    B. Coronary artery disease (CAD)
    C. Peripheral arterial disease (PAD)
    D. Abdominal aortic aneurysm (AAA)
    E. Diabetes mellitus (DM)
3. Assess patient for modifiable risk factors for CVD and initiate a treatment plan for risk factor reduction
4. Interpret results of laboratory tests
5. Monitor patient's ability to follow the treatment plan
6. Monitor patient's response to treatment plan for CVD risk factor reduction, TLC, dietary and medication regimens

Intervention

1. Treat dyslipidemias considering KDOQI clinical practice guidelines (2003 or most recent update) and Adult Treatment Panel III (ATP III) Guidelines (2003 or most recent update)
    A. CKD patients are in the highest risk category
    B. Evaluate patient for dyslipidemias at presentation with CKD, status change, and at least annually
    C. Consider initiating pharmacotherapy 3 months after TLC initiated if not within target range
    D. Cardiovascular risk factor identification and reduction should begin with diagnosis of CKD
2. Order diagnostic studies; evaluate frequency of laboratory testing
3. Adjust medication regimen as appropriate, based on patient response
4. Adjust diet prescription based on assessment of patient
5. Collaborate with and provide support and education for primary care providers, diabetes nurse educators, and other health care professionals to enhance patient screening and early referral

References

Expert Panel on Detection, Evaluation and Treatment of High Blood Cholesterol in Adults (ATP III Guidelines). (2003). Executive summary of the third report of the national cholesterol education program (NCEP) expert panel on detection, evaluation, and treatment of high blood cholesterol in adults (Adult Treatment Panel III). *Journal of the American Medical Association, 285*, 2486-2497.

National Kidney Foundation. (2003b). K/DOQI clinical practice guidelines for managing dyslipidemias in chronic kidney disease. *American Journal of Kidney Diseases, 41*(4)(Suppl. 3), S1-S91.

Cardiovascular risk factor identification and reduction should begin with diagnosis

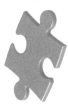

Fluid Balance and Congestive Heart Failure

Patient Outcomes

The patient will maintain euvolemia.

The patient will be free of signs and symptoms of congestive heart failure (CHF).

The patient with CKD will demonstrate knowledge about risks, prevention, and treatment related to fluid management.

Nursing Care

Assessment

1. Assess the patient's
   A. Weight
   B. Blood pressure (BP) (lying, sitting, standing)
   C. Apical and peripheral pulses (quality, rate, rhythm)
   D. Heart sounds
   E. Respiratory rate and quality
   F. Breath sounds
   G. Neck vein distention, jugular venous pressure
   H. Peripheral edema
   I. Skin turgor and mucous membranes
   J. Sodium intake
   K. Adherence to dietary and medication regimens
   L. Response to diuretics
   M. If patient receiving acute care

2. Assess intake and output; include any fluid losses related to draining wounds, nasogastric tube, fever, diarrhea, diaphoresis, hyperventilation

3. Assess the patient for
   A. Symptoms of orthostasis (e.g., dizziness, lightheadedness)
   B. Shortness of breath, dyspnea on exertion, orthopnea

4. Review laboratory test results
   A. Blood urea nitrogen
   B. Serum creatinine
   C. Electrolytes
   D. Hemoglobin
   E. Hematocrit

5. Review results of electrocardiogram (EKG), chest x-ray, and other diagnostic studies

6. Assess the patient's understanding of fluid management

Intervention

1. Collaborate with health care professionals including nephrologist, advanced practice nurse, and renal dietitian in determining appropriate fluid, dietary, and medication regimens

2. Administer diuretics as ordered

3. Administer oxygen as ordered

Assess the patient's understanding of fluid management

Fluid Balance

4. Administer and monitor fluids according to prescribed treatment plan
5. Treat anemia, if present
6. Encourage adherence to prescribed fluid and dietary regimens
7. Encourage adherence to medication regimen
8. Identify resources to assist patient to achieve fluid management goals
9. Initiate or request consultations and referrals as appropriate

Patient Teaching

Before teaching begins, consider health literacy and individualize the approach by considering patient's cultural and health beliefs, preferences, and wishes

1. Educate patient regarding
   A. Kidney function and its relationship to fluid balance
   B. Blood pressure and its relationship to fluid balance
   C. Signs and symptoms of hypervolemia and hypovolemia
   D. Causes, signs, and symptoms of cardiac alterations (including CHF) related to fluid balance
   E. Diet and fluid prescription, including sodium intake
   F. Thirst management

Advanced Practice Nursing Care

(In addition to items outlined above)

Monitor the patient's response to the treatment plan

Assessment

1. Estimate the patient's glomerular filtration rate (GFR) using a prediction equation at each health encounter
2. Interpret results of diagnostic studies (e.g., laboratory tests, EKG, chest x-ray, echocardiogram)
3. Monitor the patient's response to the treatment plan
   A. Monitor patients treated with nonpotassium-sparing diuretics for volume depletion (e.g., hypotension, decreased GFR, and hypokalemia)
   B. Monitor patients treated with potassium-sparing diuretics for volume depletion and hyperkalemia
   C. Monitor patients treated with angiotensin-converting enzyme (ACE) inhibitors or angiotensin receptor blockers (ARBs) for hypotension, decreased GFR, and hyperkalemia
   D. After initiation or increase in dose of diuretic, ACE inhibitor, or ARB, monitor BP, GFR, and serum potassium
   E. After BP is at goal and dose of medication is stable, monitor BP, GFR, and serum potassium at intervals based on the type of diuretic, baseline GFR, and baseline serum potassium
4. Monitor patient's ability to follow the treatment plan

Reference

Nielsen, S., Knepper, M.A., Kwon, T.H., & Frokiaer, J. (2004). Regulation of water balance. In B.M. Brenner (Ed.), *Brenner and Rector's the kidney* (7th ed., Vol. 1), 109-134. Philadelphia: Saunders.

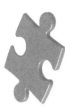

Glycemic Control

Patient Outcomes

The patient will achieve and maintain blood glucose levels in acceptable range.

There will be a slowing of progression of complications of diabetes mellitus (DM) including retinopathy, neuropathy, nephropathy, and cardiovascular disease.

The patient will demonstrate knowledge of glucose self-management.

Nursing Care

Assessment

1. Perform a health history
   A. Address family history of diabetes mellitus (DM)
2. Assess the patient's
   A. Weight, body mass index (BMI), waist circumference
   B. Dietary intake
   C. Ability to follow prescribed diet and medication regimens, and to identify barriers
   D. Therapeutic lifestyle changes (TLC), including smoking, alcohol consumption, and exercise
3. Assess the patient for
   A. Weight loss or gain
   B. Presence of anorexia, nausea, vomiting, diarrhea, or constipation
   C. Gastrointestinal conditions affecting appetite and ability to absorb nutrients
4. Assess the patient's dietary habits and cultural or ethnic values regarding food preferences, eating patterns, economic factors, health literacy
5. Review laboratory test results including blood urea nitrogen (BUN), creatinine, blood glucose, fasting blood glucose, postprandial blood glucose, glycosylated hemoglobin (HbA1c) levels, and presence of microalbuminuria or proteinuria at least annually
6. Evaluate and manage inflammation and nutrition
   A. Collect data to establish baseline nutritional and inflammatory state including, but not limited to, albumin, body mass index, evaluation of dietary intake, ferritin, or subjective global assessment
7. Review results of patient's blood glucose self-monitoring
8. Assess the patient's knowledge and understanding of glycemic control

Intervention

Interventions will be implemented, aimed at slowing the progression of the disease.

1. Collaborate with health care providers such as nephrologist, advanced practice nurse, dietitian, primary care provider, and/or diabetic treatment center in planning appropriate TLC, dietary prescription, and medication regimen
2. Test blood glucose levels as prescribed
3. Ensure medications are taken as prescribed
4. Encourage dietary adherence to prescribed regimen and identify barriers
   A. Assist the patient to incorporate the prescribed diet based on ethnic and/or cultural preferences

Evaluate and manage inflammation and nutrition

Glycemic Control

5. Encourage physical activity and promote food choices that facilitate moderate weight loss or prevent weight gain
6. Identify resources to assist patient to achieve glucose goals
7. Request or initiate consultations and referrals as appropriate

Patient Teaching

Before teaching begins, consider health literacy and individualize the approach by considering patient's cultural and health beliefs, preferences, and wishes

1. Educate patient regarding
   A. Kidney function, glomerular filtration rate (GFR), and the effect of elevated blood glucose levels on kidney function and other organs
   B. Normal blood glucose levels and HbA1c
   C. Microalbuminuria or proteinuria and its effect on progression of CKD and development of CVD
   D. Symptoms of hyperglycemia and hypoglycemia
   E. Weight loss and effect on blood glucose levels
   F. TLC and effects on blood glucose levels
   G. Effect of acute illness on blood glucose levels
   H. Diet modification and prescription
   I. Self-management of blood glucose, including treatment of hyperglycemia and prevention of hypoglycemia as it relates to patient's renal function and current diet and medication regimens

Assess the patient for risk factors for development of type 2 DM

Advanced Practice Nursing Care

(In addition to items outlined above)

Assessment

1. Estimate the patient's glomerular filtration rate (GFR) using a prediction equation at each health encounter
2. Assess the patient for risk factors for development of type 2 DM
   A. Age >45
   B. Overweight (BMI >25 kg/m^2)
   C. Family history
   D. Habitual physical inactivity
   E. Race and ethnicity
   F. Previously identified impaired fasting glucose (IFG) or impaired glucose tolerance (IGT)
   G. History of gestational diabetes mellitus (GDM) or delivery of baby weighing >9 lb
   H. Hypertension
   I. High-density lipoprotein (HDL) <35 mg/dL or 0.35 g/L; or triglyceride level >250 mg/dL or 2.9 mmol/L
   J. Polycystic ovary syndrome
   K. History of vascular disease
3. Interpret results of diagnostic studies, including urine microalbuminuria or proteinuria and patient's blood glucose self-monitoring results
4. Monitor patient's ability to follow the treatment plan
5. Monitor patient's response to the treatment plan

Glycemic Control

Intervention

1. Prescribe and treat DM considering the most current recommendations from the American Diabetes Association
   A. Diet
   B. TLC
   C. Blood glucose monitoring and self-management
   D. Medications
2. Order diagnostic studies as appropriate
3. Adjust medication regimen as appropriate, based on patient's response
4. Adjust diet prescription based on assessment of patient's response
5. Collaborate with primary care providers, diabetes nurse educators, and other health care professionals to enhance patient screening and early referral

References

American Diabetes Association. (2004c). Nutrition principles and recommendations in diabetes. *Diabetes Care, 27*(Suppl. 1), S36-S46.

American Diabetes Association. (2010). Diagnosis and classification of diabetes mellitus. *Diabetes Care, 33*(S62-69). doi: 10.2337/dcro-S062.

American Diabetes Association. (2004b). Nephropathy in diabetes. *Diabetes Care, 27*(Suppl. 1), S79-S83.

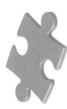

Hypertension

Patient Outcomes

The patient will achieve and maintain blood pressure (BP) within the targeted range.

The patient will demonstrate a reduction in modifiable risk for cardiovascular disease (CVD).

The patient will demonstrate knowledge and self-management strategies of hypertension and its relationship to CKD and CVD.

Nursing Care

Assessment

1. Measure BP at each health encounter (lying, sitting, standing)
   A. Measure BP at least two times and calculate the average of the readings
   B. Compare to the targeted goal of <130/80 mmHg and previous readings
2. Perform a health history
   A. Address family history of hypertension (HTN) and other risk factors for HTN and CVD (Chobanian et al., 2004)
3. Conduct a physical assessment
   A. Weight
   B. Respiratory rate and quality
   C. Heart sounds
   D. Breath sounds
   E. Dependent and peripheral edema

Hypertension

   F. Neck vein distention, jugular venous pressure
   G. Ability to follow prescribed treatment regimen
     (1) identify barriers to self-management
     (2) recommended therapeutic lifestyle changes (TLC)
       a. dietary modifications and medication regimen
       b. smoking cessation and alcohol reduction
4. Review appropriate data
   A. Home BP record
   B. Review laboratory test results
   C. Review results of electrocardiogram (EKG), chest x-rays, other diagnostic studies
5. Assess the patient's understanding of prescription regimen

Intervention

Interventions will be implemented to control hypertension, and modifiable risk factors will be reduced

1. Collaborate with other health care professionals such as nephrologist, advanced practice nurse, primary care provider, and dietitian in planning appropriate BP goals and therapeutic regimen
2. Encourage adherence to prescribed medication regimen
   A. Perform medication review each health encounter
3. Encourage adherence to TLC and dietary modifications
4. Identify resources to assist patient to achieve goals of blood pressure control
5. Request or initiate consultations and referrals as appropriate

Patient Teaching

Before teaching begins, consider health literacy and individualize the approach by considering patient's cultural and health beliefs, preferences, and wishes

1. Teach the patient to measure and record BP
2. Instruct the patient regarding
   A. Management of HTN
   B. Prescribed antihypertensive medications
   C. Prescribed dietary modifications
   D. Recommended TLC
   E. Proper BP measurement technique
   F. HTN and risk of CKD and the relationship between HTN and CKD
   G. Causes, signs, and symptoms of cardiac alterations related to HTN
   H. Signs and symptoms of hypotension
   I. Reading and comprehending food labels.

Advanced Practice Nursing Care

(In addition to items outlined above)

Assessment

1. Ascertain the presence and stage of CKD; if possible identify cause of CKD as follows
   A. Estimate the patient's glomerular filtration rate (GFR) using a prediction equation
   B. Determine the presence and level of proteinuria/microalbuminuria
   C. Examine microscopic urine sediment
   D. If appropriate, order and interpret renal ultrasound
2. Ascertain the presence of CVD or CVD risk factors
   A. If appropriate, obtain 12-lead EKG

Assess the patient's understanding of prescription regimen

Hypertension

B. If appropriate, obtain laboratory studies such as fasting lipid panel, fasting and postprandial serum glucose

C. Calculate body mass index (BMI) at annual health examination

D. Measure waist circumference

3. Assess for signs and symptoms of other chronic disease processes

4. Monitor for complications and side effects of pharmacologic therapy

5. Monitor adherence to treatment plan and barriers to adherence

Intervention

1. Recommend dietary modifications and TLC as adjunct therapy in the treatment of HTN considering the KDOQI clinical practice guidelines (2004 or most recent updates) and JNC VII (2003 or most recent updates) as follows

   A. DASH Diet (CKD Stages 1–2); modified DASH Diet (CKD Stages 3–4)

   B. Implement strategies aimed at weight loss, if obese, or maintenance of desirable body weight

   C. Encourage patient to engage in an exercise and physical activity program

   D. Moderation of alcohol intake

   E. If patient smokes, establish smoking cessation strategies with patient

2. Prescribe pharmacologic therapy (preferred agent) based on the type of kidney disease, level of proteinuria, and BP considering KDOQI clinical practice guidelines (2004 or most recent updates) and JNC VII (2003 or most recent updates) as follows

   A. Diabetic kidney disease

      (1) preferred agents – angiotensin-converting enzyme (ACE) inhibitor or angiotensin receptor blocker (ARB)

      (2) diuretic, then beta-blocker or calcium-channel blocker

   B. Nondiabetic kidney disease with spot urine protein-to-creatinine ratio >200 mg/g

      (1) preferred agents – ACE inhibitor or ARB

      (2) diuretic, then beta-blocker or calcium-channel blocker

   C. Nondiabetic kidney disease with spot urine protein-to-creatinine ratio <200 mg/g

      (1) diuretic preferred, then ACE inhibitor, ARB, beta-blocker, or calcium-channel blocker

3. Order laboratory and diagnostic studies as appropriate

4. Adjust medication regimen as appropriate, based on patient response

5. Initiate evaluation of causes for secondary HTN, if indicated

6. Collaborate with and provide support and education for primary care providers and other health care professionals to enhance patient screening for CKD and early referral

Implement strategies aimed at prevention and slowing progression of kidney disease

References

Chobanian, A.V., Bakris, G.L., Black, H.R., Cushman, W.C., Green, L.A., Izzo, J.L., Jr., Jones, D.W., Materson, B.J., Oparil, S., Wright, J.T., Jr., & Rocella, E.J. National Heart, Lung, and Blood Institute Joint National Committee on Prevention, Detection, Evaluation, and Treatment of High Blood Pressure. (2004). The seventh report of the Joint National Committee on Prevention, Detection, Evaluation, and Treatment of High Blood Pressure: The JNC 7 report. *Journal of the American Medical Association, 289*(19), 2560-2572.

National Kidney Foundation. (2004). K/DOQI clinical practice guidelines on hypertension and antihypertensive agents in chronic kidney disease. *American Journal of Kidney Diseases, 43*(5)(Suppl. 1), S1-S290.

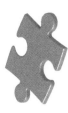

Nutrition and Metabolic Control

Patient Outcomes

The patient will achieve and maintain ideal desired body weight, nutritional status, and electrolyte and metabolic balance.

The patient will demonstrate knowledge of nutritional requirements to promote health in chronic kidney disease (CKD).

Nursing Care

Assessment

1. Perform a health history
2. Assess the patient's
   A. Weight and body mass index (BMI)
   B. Muscle mass and strength
   C. Edema
   D. Nutrient intake
   E. Lifestyle habits including smoking, alcohol consumption, and exercise frequency
   F. Urine for microalbuminuria or proteinuria
   G. Ability to follow diet and medication regimens
3. Assess patient for
   A. Weight loss or gain over past week, 6 months, or year
   B. Gastrointestinal conditions affecting appetite and ability to absorb nutrients; presence of anorexia, nausea, vomiting, diarrhea, or constipation
   C. Food allergies
4. Assess psychosocial factors that contribute to ability to follow diet and medication prescriptions
5. Assess the patient's dietary habits and cultural or ethnic values regarding food preferences, eating patterns, economic factors
6. Review laboratory test results including blood urea nitrogen (BUN), creatinine, albumin, prealbumin, calcium, phosphorous, magnesium, potassium, sodium, hemoglobin, and hematocrit
7. Assess patient's knowledge and understanding of nutrition and metabolic control

Intervention

1. Collaborate with health care professionals including nephrologist, advanced practice nurse, primary care provider, dietitian, and social worker in planning appropriate dietary and medication regimens
2. Ensure medications are administered as prescribed to treat gastrointestinal conditions affecting appetite
3. Encourage dietary adherence according to prescribed regimen and help the patient incorporate the prescribed diet to satisfy food preferences and lifestyle
4. Encourage physical activity and promote food choices that facilitate moderate weight loss or at least prevent weight gain
5. Identify resources to assist patient to achieve dietary goals
6. Request or initiate consultations and referrals as appropriate
7. Evaluate and treat proteinuria

Identify resources to assist patient to achieve dietary goals

Nutrition and Metabolic Control

Patient Teaching

Before teaching begins, consider health literacy and individualize the approach by considering patient's cultural and health beliefs, preferences, and wishes

1. Educate patient regarding
   A. Kidney function and its effect on nutrient intake
   B. Gastrointestinal conditions affecting appetite
   C. Signs and symptoms of protein-energy malnutrition
   D. Signs and symptoms of the following
      (1) volume overload or depletion
      (2) hypo- or hyperkalemia
      (3) hypo- or hypercalcemia
      (4) hypo- or hyperphosphatemia
      (5) hypo- or hypermagnesemia
   E. Diet prescription and nutritional requirements including
      (1) caloric intake
      (2) protein requirements
      (3) minerals
      (4) fluid
   F. Ideal body weight and BMI
   G. Therapeutic lifestyle changes (TLC)
   H. Vitamins and dietary supplements
   I. Management of nutritional status and electrolyte and metabolic balance as they relate to the patient's current diet, fluid, and medications

Advanced Practice Nursing Care

(In addition to items outlined above)

Assessment

1. Estimate the patient's glomerular filtration rate (GFR) using a prediction equation each health encounter
2. As GFR declines, assess patient for protein-energy malnutrition. Monitor for every stage, but assess at Stage 3
   A. Serum albumin or prealbumin initial visit
   B. Thereafter, monitor 3–6 months or more frequently if warranted
   C. In collaboration with the renal dietitian, assess edema-free actual body weight, percent standard (National Health and Nutrition Examination Survey II [NHANES II]) body weight, or subjective global assessment
   D. Normalized protein nitrogen appearance (nPNA) as needed
3. Interpret results of laboratory tests
4. Monitor patient's ability to follow the treatment plan
5. Monitor patient's response to treatment plan

Intervention

1. Implement strategies aimed at prevention and, if occurs, treat malnutrition, electrolyte and metabolic imbalances considering recommendations from the KDOQI clinical practice guidelines (2000 or most recent update)
   A. Diet prescription and nutritional requirements
   B. TLC
   C. Medications
2. Order laboratory tests and diagnostic studies as appropriate
3. Adjust medication regimen as appropriate, based on patient response
4. Adjust diet prescription based on assessment of patient

As GFR declines, assess patient for protein-energy malnutrition

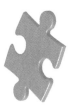

Nutrition and Metabolic Control

References

National Kidney Foundation. (2002). K/DOQI clinical practice guidelines for chronic kidney disease: Evaluation, classification and stratification. *American Journal of Kidney Diseases, 39*(2)(Suppl. 1), S1-S266.

National Kidney Foundation. (2004). K/DOQI clinical practice guidelines on hypertension and antihypertensive agents in chronic kidney disease. *American Journal of Kidney Diseases, 43*(5)(Suppl. 1), S1-S290.

National Kidney Foundation. (2000b). K/DOQI clinical practice guidelines for nutrition in chronic renal failure. *American Journal of Kidney Diseases, 35*(6)(Suppl. 2), S1-S140. Erratum in: (2001). *American Journal of Kidney Diseases, 38*(4), 917.

Preparation for Replacement Therapy

Patient Outcomes

The patient will demonstrate knowledge of chronic kidney disease (CKD) and its implications.

The patient will participate in the decision-making process for treatment modality selection.

The patient will have a functioning permanent dialysis access prior to initiation of dialysis.

The patient will have completed evaluation for kidney transplant if appropriate.

The patient will convert to hepatitis B antibody-positive status.

Pediatric Patient Outcomes

The parent(s) and primary caregiver(s) will demonstrate knowledge of chronic kidney disease, its systemic effects, and the treatment required to control the effects of declining kidney function.

The child will participate in his/her care as appropriate as determined by the health care team members, parents, and child and will be consistent with the child's capacity to participate. Ultimately, the child should be ready to take responsibility for his/her care as an adult.

The parent(s) will participate in the development of the child's plan of care.

Nursing Care

Assessment

1. Assess the patient for signs and symptoms of uremia and for any absolute indications for initiation of kidney replacement therapy
2. In collaboration with the interdisciplinary health care team, patient, and patient family, assess patient's suitability for specific dialysis modalities
3. In collaboration with the health care team, assess the patient's suitability for kidney transplantation (e.g., physical condition, psychosocial condition)
4. Assess patient's coping abilities
5. Evaluate the patient's ability and readiness to learn
   A. Physical condition
   B. Ability to concentrate

Preparation for Replacement Therapy

    C. Psychological status

    D. Developmental stage

    E. Degree of motivation

    F. Literacy level

    G. Preferred method of learning

6. Identify potential barriers to learning (e.g., cultural beliefs and practices, language, literacy level, age, environment)
7. Review laboratory values
    A. Blood urea nitrogen (BUN) and creatinine
    B. Hemoglobin and hematocrit
    C. Albumin
    D. Phosphorus
    E. Hepatitis B antigen and antibody
8. Assess the patient's current level of knowledge related to
    A. Etiology of CKD and its implications
    B. Prognosis and expected progression of disease
    C. CKD treatment plan
    D. Signs and symptoms of uremia
    E. Dialysis treatment options
    F. Access for dialysis
    G. Hepatitis
    H. Kidney transplantation

For the pediatric patient: In conjunction with the parents, determine the child's current level of knowledge, ability to learn, and the appropriate level of involvement in the learning process.

Provide information regarding replacement therapy

Intervention

1. Collaborate with the interdisciplinary team, including the patient, to develop a treatment and teaching plan that takes into consideration time until initiation of replacement therapy
2. For pediatric patients: develop a plan of care that includes the parent(s) and child as appropriate. Encourage parent(s) to identify patient and family-centered goals
3. Encourage the patient to preserve upper extremity or other potential access sites, if indicated, for hemodialysis access (no IVs or venipunctures)
4. Administer hepatitis B immunizations as prescribed
5. Offer support and reassurance, encouraging verbalization of questions or concerns
6. Identify resources to assist patient with selection of and adjustment to replacement therapy
7. Request or initiate consultations and referrals as appropriate

Patient Teaching

Before teaching begins, consider health literacy and individualize the approach by considering patient's cultural and health beliefs, preferences, and wishes

1. Provide information regarding replacement therapy. Use techniques and materials appropriate for the patient's developmental stage, culture, and disabilities
2. Identify members of the health care team and their roles
3. Dialysis modality education should include, but not be limited to
    A. Modality types
        (1) hemodialysis
        (2) peritoneal dialysis
        (3) kidney transplantation
        (4) conservative management with palliative care

Preparation for Replacement Therapy

B. Dialysis process and procedures
C. Access placement
D. Treatment medications
E. Advantages and disadvantages of each modality
F. Expected outcomes
G. Complications
H. Lifestyle adaptation
I. Rehabilitation potential
J. Financial considerations

4. Transplant education should include, but not be limited to
A. Definitions and types of transplants
B. Evaluation process
C. Surgical procedure
D. Advantages and disadvantages
E. Expected outcomes
F. Lifestyle adaptation
G. Rehabilitation potential
H. Financial considerations

5. Describe signs and symptoms of uremia as well as absolute indications for initiation of dialysis

6. Discuss temporary hemodialysis access if needed

7. Explain rationale for hepatitis surveillance

8. Provide information regarding hepatitis immunization

Describe signs and symptoms of uremia

9. Instruct patient to notify health care team of new medications, both prescribed and over-the-counter

10. Reinforce teaching as necessary, using varied teaching approaches, return demonstrations, verbal and written feedback

11. Include family or other support persons in the education process

Advanced Practice Nursing Care
(In addition to items outlined above)

Assessment

1. Estimate the patient's GFR using a prediction equation at each health encounter
2. Monitor patient for signs and symptoms of progression of CKD and need to initiate replacement therapy
3. Interpret results of laboratory tests as related to the progression of CKD
4. Monitor patient's ability to follow prescribed treatment plan
5. Assess patient for placement of permanent dialysis access
6. Monitor response to hepatitis B immunization as recommended by the Centers for Disease Control and Prevention (CDC)

Intervention

1. Collaborate with and provide support and education for primary care providers, diabetes nurse educators, and other health care professionals to enhance patient screening and early referral
2. Refer for dialysis access placement as appropriate
3. Refer for kidney transplant evaluation as appropriate
4. Initiate dialysis or refer to a dialysis unit for initiation of treatment when appropriate
5. If patient chooses no treatment, refer to appropriate individuals to facilitate palliative care
6. Order hepatitis B and other immunizations as appropriate
7. Adjust treatment plan as necessary, based on patient response

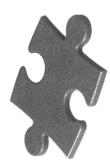

Nephrology Nursing Care

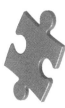

Anemia

Patient Outcomes

The patient will achieve and maintain hemoglobin (Hb) and hematocrit (Hct) within the targeted range.

The patient will demonstrate knowledge concerning anemia and its implications.

The patient will demonstrate knowledge concerning treatment options, including benefits and risks.

Nursing Care

Assessment

1. Assess the patient's
   A. Weight
   B. Blood pressure and heart rate
   C. Respiratory rate and quality
   D. Skin and mucous membranes

Anemia

E. Adherence to medication regimen

F. Volume status

2. Assess the patient for signs and symptoms of anemia

A. Angina, hypotension, tachycardia, shortness of breath

B. Decreased energy and activity levels

C. Anorexia

D. Decreased sense of well-being and quality of life

E. Decreased skeletal muscle function and weakness

F. Impaired sexual function

G. Impaired cognition and mental sluggishness

H. Sleep dysfunction including restless legs (RLS)

I. Depression

3. Review laboratory test results

A. Blood urea nitrogen, serum creatinine, and estimated glomerular filtration rate

B. Complete blood count (CBC) including red blood cell indices (mean corpuscular hemoglobin [MCH], mean corpuscular volume [MCV], mean corpuscular hemoglobin concentration [MCHC]), white blood cell count, and differential and platelet count

C. Iron profile (i.e., iron, ferritin, total iron binding capacity [TIBC], transferrin saturation [TSAT], and reticulocyte hemoglobin content [CHr])

D. Folate and B_{12} levels

E. Albumin

Assess patient for causes of anemia

4. Assess patient for causes of anemia

A. Blood loss

B. Iron or vitamin deficiencies

C. Inflammation or infection

D. Secondary hyperparathyroidism

E. Medications

F. Coexisting medical conditions

G. Malnutrition

H. Hospitalization

I. Vascular access procedure

J Catheter as vascular access

K. Mode of dialysis

5. Assess patient's understanding of anemia

Intervention

1. Collaborate with health care professionals including physician and advanced practice provider to develop and use an anemia management protocol

2. Ensure medications are administered as prescribed, including iron supplements, vitamins, and erythropoeisis-stimulating agents (ESAs)

3. Monitor response to therapy, including

A. Hemoglobin and hematocrit trends

B. Iron profile

C. Sense of well-being

(*Frequency of monitoring is based on therapy response and goals*)

4. Monitor blood pressure and report elevations to physician or advanced practice provider

5. Monitor patient for potential causes of hyporesponse to anemia treatment and report to physician or advanced practice provider

A. Inadequate erythropoiesis-stimulating agent (ESA) dose

Anemia

B. Iron deficiency
C. Infection or inflammation
D. Blood loss
E. Secondary hyperparathyroidism
F. Vitamin deficiency
G. Cancer
H. Malnutrition
I. Inadequate dialysis dose
J. Medications
K. Posthospitalization
L. Vascular access procedure
M. Presence of catheter

6. Encourage adherence to treatment and medication regimens
7. Identify resources to assist patient to achieve goals of anemia management
8. Request or initiate consultations or referrals as appropriate

Patient Teaching

Before education begins, consider health literacy and individualize the approach by considering the patient's cultural and health beliefs, preferences, and wishes

1. Educate the patient regarding
   A. Kidney function and its relationship to anemia
   B. Signs and symptoms of anemia
   C. Consequences of anemia, including left ventricular hypertrophy (LVH)
   D. Diagnostic tests used to evaluate anemia
   E. Signs of gastrointestinal bleeding
      (1) hematemesis
      (2) tarry stool
   F. Iron and vitamin levels and their effects on erythropoiesis
   G. Management of anemia, including administration of iron and ESAs
      (1) benefits
      (2) risks
2. Instruct patient regarding information to report to the nurse or health care team, including changes in symptoms and signs of bleeding

> **Monitor patient for potential causes of hyporesponse to anemia management**

Advanced Practice Nursing Care

(In addition to items outlined above)

Assessment

1. Interpret results of diagnostic studies (e.g., laboratory tests, electrocardiogram [EKG], echocardiogram)
2. Initiate an anemia workup per current KDOQI Clinical Practice Guidelines for facility anemia management protocol
3. Monitor patient's ability to follow the treatment plan
4. Monitor patient's response to treatment plan
5. Monitor BP and adjust therapy as need
6. Monitor patient for potential causes of hyporesponse to anemia management

Intervention

1. Treat anemia following the most current KDOQI clinical practice guidelines (2006)
   A. Establish target hemoglobin (National Kidney Foundation, 2007a)
   B. Initiate an anemia workup

Anemia

    C. Develop and use an anemia management protocol
2. Order laboratory tests and diagnostic studies as appropriate
3. Adjust medication regimen based on patient response
4. Adjust BP medications as indicated for increased BP
5. Consult hematology if cause of hyporesponse is not evident
6. Consult oncology if treating patient with cancer

References

National Kidney Foundation. (2000a). K/DOQI clinical practice guidelines for anemia of chronic kidney disease: Update 2000. *American Journal of Kidney Diseases, 37*(1)(Suppl. 1), S182-S238.

National Kidney Foundation. (2006a). KDOQI clinical practice guidelines and clinical practice recommendations for anemia of chronic kidney disease. *American Journal of Kidney Diseases, 47*(5)(Suppl. 3), S1-S145.

National Kidney Foundation. (2007a). KDOQI clinical practice guidelines for anemia of chronic kidney disease: 2007 update of hemoglobin target. *American Journal of Kidney Diseases, 50*(3), 471-530.

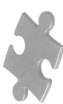

Bowel Function

Patient Outcome

The patient will establish a desired bowel elimination pattern.

Nursing Care

Assessment

1. Determine usual bowel pattern, past and current history of bowel problems
2. Assess food habits and tolerances
3. Review diet, fluid, and medication prescriptions, and assess patient's adherence to the treatment regimen
4. Assess use of over-the-counter medications and treatments (e.g., laxatives and enemas)
5. Assess physical activity level
6. Auscultate for bowel sounds
7. Assess characteristics of stools
    A. Color
    B. Consistency
    C. Frequency
    D. Evidence of bleeding
8. Assess for conditions that may make patient reluctant to have bowel movements
    A. Hemorrhoids
    B. Perianal excoriation
    C. Pain during defecation
    D. Embarrassment related to ostomy or incontinence
    E. Disruption of routine
    F. Pain or difficulty with walking
    G. Embarrassment of dependence on others for toileting

Intervention

1. Collaborate with interdisciplinary team to help patient find best regimen for bowel elimination, which may include
    A. Diet changes

Bowel Function

   B. Stool softeners
   C. Laxatives
   D. Medications that promote gastric emptying
   E. Altered doses of other medications
2. Reinforce inclusion of dietary fiber
3. Encourage fluid intake within prescribed limits
4. Encourage physical activity
5. Consult clinical specialists as needed, for ostomy, perianal excoriation, or hemorrhoid management

Patient Teaching

Before teaching begins, consider health literacy and individualize the approach by considering patient's cultural and health beliefs, preferences, and wishes

1. Discuss reasons for bowel dysfunction, including the potential for medication-induced constipation or diarrhea
2. Collaborate with health care team to provide appropriate education regarding diet, fluids, medications, activity, and skin care
3. Instruct the patient in the use of prescribed bowel management aids and the consequences of long-term laxative use
4. Advise patient to report any changes in color or consistency of stool
5. Discuss implications of constipation with patient undergoing peritoneal dialysis
6. Discuss hygiene in relation to the prevention of perianal infection and potential for cross-contamination to urine, vagina, catheters, and wounds
7. Discuss implications of diarrhea with the posttransplant patient
8. Discuss implications of diarrhea on dry weight with the hemodialysis patient
9. Warn dialysis patients about the danger of using phosphate-containing enemas such as the Fleet enema

Warn dialysis patients about the danger of using phosphate-containing enemas

Advanced Practice Nursing Care

(In addition to items outlined above)

Assessment

1. Assess the patient's response to the current treatment regimen

Intervention

1. Adjust medications (laxatives, antidiarrheal agents, analgesics, and other drugs that impact bowel function) and diet (fiber, dairy products, etc.) as patient condition indicates
2. Collaborate with other health care providers as needed

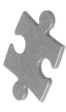

Chronic Kidney Disease – Mineral and Bone Disorder (CKD-MBD)

Patient Outcomes

The patient will maintain mineral biochemical parameters and acid-base balance within the targeted range.

The patient will be free of disability related to bone disease, calcific cardiovascular abnormalities, and other soft tissue calcification.

CKD-MBD

The patient will demonstrate knowledge of CKD-MBD and its complications including bone disease, calcific cardiovascular abnormalities, and soft tissue calcification.

The patient will demonstrate knowledge of his or her role in prevention, management, and progression of CKD-MBD.

Nursing Care

Assessment

1. Assess the patient's
   A. Muscle strength, gait, and range of motion, noting limitations in movement
   B. Height or linear growth (pediatric patient)
   C. Joints for enlargement, swelling, stiffness, and tenderness
   D. Bone pain
   E. Skin for local tissue injury, macules, papules, or pruritis
   F. Eyes for visible irritation and local inflammation
   G. Extremities for presence and quality of pulse and vascular insufficiency
   H. Blood pressure and heart rate (lying, sitting, standing) and heart rate

2. Assess the patient for
   A. Clinical risk factors for fracture
      (1) advancing age
      (2) female gender
      (3) Caucasian race
      (4) low body weight (less than 58 kg)
      (5) previous adult fracture
      (6) parental history of hip fracture
      (7) current or history of cigarette smoking
      (8) excessive alcohol use
      (9) rheumatoid arthritis
      (10) glucocorticosteroid therapy
   B. Other risk factors for fracture
      (1) Vitamin D deficiency
      (2) Recurrent falls or use of walking aids
      (3) Dementia or poor health/frailty
   C. History of injuries or falls, the progression of healing, and the potential for new injuries
   D. Ability to follow diet, medication, and treatment regimens
   E. Financial constraints in meeting dietary and medication regimens

3. Assess the patient's environment for potential hazards

4. Review laboratory test results, magnitude of abnormality, and trend
   A. Serum calcium
   B. Phosphorous
   C. Parathyroid hormone (PH)
   D. Alkaline phosphatase
   E. CO_2
   F. 25-OH vitamin D
   G. Aluminum

5. Review results of diagnostic tests
   A. Lateral abdominal radiograph
   B. Electrocardiogram (EKG)

CKD-MBD

C. Echocardiogram
6. Assess patient's understanding of CKD-MBD

Intervention

1. Collaborate with nephrologist, advanced practice nurse, dietitian, social worker, and patient in planning appropriate dietary, medication, and treatment regimens
2. Maintain mineral biochemical parameters in the target range
   A. Correct dialysate calcium level
   B. Phosphate binder
   C. Limit dietary phosphorous
   D. Delivery of dialysis prescription
3. Ensure medications are administered as prescribed
   A. Phosphate binder
   B. Calcium supplement
   C. Calcimimetic
   D. Alkali salts
   E. Vitamin D
4. Monitor for side effects of treatments
5. Encourage adherence to prescribed dietary and medication regimens
6. Collaborate with social worker to assure a safe home environment and financial assistance as needed for dietary and medication regimens
7. Collaborate with physical therapy for recommended aids for mobility as appropriate
8. Identify resources to assist patient to achieve goals of CKD-MBD and prevention of complications
9. Initiate and request consultations and referrals as appropriate

Patient Teaching

Before teaching begins, consider health literacy and individualize the approach by considering patient's cultural and health beliefs, preferences, and wishes

1. Educate the patient regarding
   A. Kidney function and its relationship to CKD-MBD
   B. Dialysis prescription and its relationship to CKD-MBD
   C. Consequences of alterations in mineral biochemical parameters
      (1) bone disease
      (2) calcific cardiovascular abnormalities
      (3) soft tissue calcification
   D. Signs and symptoms of
      (1) bone disease
      (2) calcific cardiovascular abnormalities
      (3) soft tissue calcification
      (4) hypo- and hyperphosphatemia
      (5) hypo- and hypercalcemia
   E. Timing of medications related to meals
   F. Reduction of mobility hazards in the home and work environment
   G. Exercises to maintain strength and mobility
2. Instruct the patient regarding information to report to the nurse or health care team, including changes in ability to exercise or mobility, falls or injuries, and pain

Maintain mineral biochemical parameters in the target range

CKD-MBD

Advanced Practice Nursing Care

(In addition to items outlined above)

Assessment

1. Monitor mineral biochemical parameters and trend
2. Monitor patient's ability to follow the treatment plan, efficacy, and side effects
   A. Diet
   B. Medications
   C. Exercise program
3. Interpret results of diagnostic studies
4. Monitor for symptoms of bone disease, calcific cardiovascular abnormalities, and other soft tissue calcification
5. Identify patients with CKD-MBD that may need referral for bone biopsy
   A. Unexplained fractures
   B. Persistent bone pain
   C. Unexplained hypophosphatemia
   D. Unexplained hypercalcemia
   E. Possible aluminum toxicity

Intervention

1. Treat disorders of CKD-MBD following the KDOQI clinical practice guidelines (2003 or most recent updates) and the KDIGO clinical practice guidelines (2009 or most recent update)
   A. Dietary prescription
   B. Medications
   C. Dialysis prescription
2. Order labs and frequency based on results, magnitude of abnormality, and trends
3. Order other diagnostic test as appropriate (e.g., lateral abdominal x-ray, EKG, and echocardiogram)
4. Adjust medication regimen and diet prescription based on biochemical parameters
5. In patients with vascular calcification, use this information to guide management of CKD-MBD
6. Refer patients with CKD-MBD for bone biopsy when indicated

Adjust medication regimen and diet prescription based on biochemical parameters

References

Kidney Disease: Improving Global Outcomes. (2009). Clinical practice guidelines for the diagnosis, evaluation, prevention, and treatment of chronic kidney disease-mineral and bone disorder (CKD-MBD). *Kidney International, 76*(Suppl. 113), S1-130.

National Kidney Foundation. (2003a). KDOQI clinical practice guidelines for bone metabolism and disease in chronic kidney disease. *American Journal of Kidney Diseases, 42*(4)(Suppl. 3), S1-S201.

Uhlig, K., Berns, J., Kestenbaum, B., Kumar, R., Leonard, M., Martin, K., Sprague, S., & Goldfarb, S. (2009). US commentary on the 2009 KDIGO clinical practice guideline for diagnosis, evaluation, and treatment of CKD-mineral and bone disorder (CKD-MBD). *American Journal of Kidney Disease, 55*(5), 773-799.

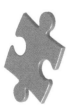

Coping

Patient Outcome

The patient will demonstrate an ability to manage CKD care utilizing effective coping strategies.

Nursing Care

Assessment

1. Assess the patient's
   A. Quality of life, including mental and physical functioning; assessment instruments for chronic kidney disease (CKD) include Short Form-36 (SF-36), Kidney Disease Quality of Life (KDQOL). Specific attention should be paid to the Mental Component Score (MCS) of the SF-36
   B. Support system, both formal and informal
   C. Emotional status
      (1) History of mood disorders including major depressive disorder, bipolar disorder, dysthymic disorder
      (2) History of anxiety disorders including generalized anxiety and panic disorder
      (3) If history is positive for either depression or anxiety, further assessment can be performed using a depression assessment tool such as the Patient Health Questionnaire-9 (PHQ-9) or an anxiety assessment tool such as the General Anxiety Disorder-7 (GAD-7)
   D. Problem-solving ability and experience
   E. Appearance
   F. Presence of stress-related symptoms
   G. Perceived degree of stress
   H. Current coping techniques and previous effective coping strategies
   I. Communication patterns, including language, education, and ability to communicate effectively
   J. Lifestyle patterns
      (1) drug and alcohol use
      (2) eating habits
      (3) exercise
      (4) sleeping habits and/or problems
   K. Previous health care experiences and cultural-specific resources used, including orientation to and experience with the U.S. health care system
   L. Current and past use of medication for the management of depression, anxiety, or any other mental health issue
   M. Financial situation
2. Assess patient's understanding of the relationship between symptoms and adherence to the treatment regimen
3. Assess impact of symptoms, disease, and treatment regimen on patient's life goals
4. Assess effect of illness and treatment regimen on patient's relationships with both formal and informal support networks

Intervention

1. Encourage use of available support resources
   A. Physical
   B. Spiritual
   C. Economic
   D. Social
   E. Psychological
2. In collaboration with the patient and the interdisciplinary team, especially the social worker, develop a plan of care that reinforces and teaches positive coping mechanisms and incorporates personal strengths
3. Encourage patient to communicate feelings and concerns to the health care team and significant other, family members, or friends

Coping

4. Assist patient to identify and practice stress-reducing techniques
5. Provide opportunity for patient to meet others who have had similar experiences
6. Initiate or request referrals to agencies or organizations for special services or support as needed
   A. Vocational rehabilitation
   B. Public health agencies
   C. Social welfare agencies
   D. Nephrology patient organizations
   E. End-stage renal disease (ESRD) networks
7. Provide anticipatory guidance and counseling regarding
   A. Identified depression
   B. Anxiety
   C. Sleep issues
   D. Dependence
   E. Body image
   F. Restrictions and limitations
   G. Fear of death
   H. Changes in interpersonal relationships
   I. Finances

Patient Teaching

Before teaching begins, consider health literacy and individualize the approach by considering patient's cultural and health beliefs, preferences, and wishes

Assist patient to identify and practice stress-reducing techniques

1. Teach effective problem-solving techniques and coping strategies
2. Review expectations of treatment regimen and impact on life goals
3. Teach the patient about symptom identification and the role of adherence to the treatment regimen in managing symptoms and overall health
4. For the patient receiving live donor kidney, discuss the emotional responses related to loss of donor's kidney (see Kidney and Pancreas Transplantation: Allograft Dysfunction)

Advanced Practice Nursing Care

(In addition to items outlined above)

Assessment

1. Acknowledge fear, anxiety, and sense of loss
2. Be cognizant of possible spousal abandonment
3. Assess for depression, especially in home patient

Intervention

1. Refer to social worker for assessment, coping strategies, and financial assistance
2. Treat depression, referral to appropriate mental health professional

References

Finkelstein, F., & Finkelstein, S. (2000). Depression in chronic dialysis patients: Assessment and treatment. *Nephrology Dialysis Transplantation, 15*(12), 1911-1913.

Hays, R.D., Kallich, J.D., Mapes, D.L., Coons, S.J., Amin, N., Carter, W.B., & Kamberg, C. (1997). *Kidney disease quality of life short form (KDQOL-SF™), Version 1.3: A manual for use and scoring*, P-7994. Santa Monica, CA: RAND.

Kidney Disease Quality of Life Working Group – www.gim.med.ucla.edu/kdqol

Performance, excellence, and accountability in kidney care – www.kidneycarequality.com

Wilson, B., Spittal, J., Heidenheim, P., Herman, M., Leonard, M., Johnston, A., Lindsay, R., & Moist, L. (2006). Screening for depression in chronic hemodialysis patients: Comparison of the Beck Depression Inventory, primary nurse, and nephrology team. *Hemodialysis International, 10*(1), 35-41.

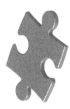

Dyslipidemia and Reduction of Cardiovascular Disease Risk Factors

Patient Outcomes

The patient will achieve and maintain lipoprotein levels within the targeted ranges.

The patient will demonstrate a reduction in modifiable risk factors for development of cardiovascular disease (CVD).

The patient will demonstrate knowledge of dyslipidemia and cardiovascular risk factor reduction.

Nursing Care

Assessment

1. Assess patient's
   A. Weight and body mass index (BMI)
   B. Blood pressure and heart rate
   C. Apical and peripheral pulses
   D. Respiratory rate and quality
   E. Peripheral edema
   F. Lifestyle habits including smoking, eating patterns, alcohol consumption, and exercise frequency
   G. Diet
   H. Medications and history of lipid-lowering medications
   I. Adherence to prescribed dietary and medication regimens
2. Assess the patient for major CVD risk factors
   A. Cigarette smoking
   B. Hypertension
   C. Obesity
   D. Low HDL (<40 mg/dL or 0.40 g/L)
   E. Family history of premature coronary heart disease (CHD)
      (1) CHD in father or brother <55 years old
      (2) CHD in mother or sister <65 years old
   F. Age
      (1) men >45 years old
      (2) women >55 years old
   G. History of myocardial infarction (MI), arrhythmia
   H. Hormone replacement therapy (HRT)
3. Assess patient for CVD risk factors
   A. Anemia
   B. Hyperhomocysteinemia
   C. Disorders of bone metabolism
   D. Volume overload
4. Review laboratory values
   A. Blood urea nitrogen and creatinine
   B. Low-density lipoprotein (LDL), total cholesterol, high-density lipoprotein (HDL)
   C. Triglycerides
   D. Hemoglobin and hematocrit
   E. Calcium, phosphorous, parathyroid hormone, and vitamin D level

Dyslipidemia – Cardiovascular

F. Homocysteine

5. Assess patient's understanding of dyslipidemia and need for reduction of cardiovascular disease risk factors

Intervention

1. Collaborate with interdisciplinary team including primary care physician in
   A. Identifying patients at risk for CVD
   B. Setting lipid goals
   C. Planning risk-factor reduction, therapeutic lifestyle changes (TLC), and medication regimen
2. Ensure medications are administered as prescribed, including aspirin, vitamins, and lipid-lowering drugs
3. Encourage adherence to TLC
4. Encourage adherence to diet, fluid restriction, dialysis treatment, and medication regimen
5. Identify resources to assist patient to achieve lipid goals
6. Request or initiate consultations and referrals as appropriate

Patient and Family Teaching

Before teaching begins, consider health literacy and individualize the approach by considering patient's cultural and health beliefs, preferences, and wishes

1. Discuss with patient
   A. Prevention and management of dyslipidemia and cardiovascular risk factor reduction as they relate to the patient's current diet, medications, and lifestyle
   B. Lipoprotein levels and effect on development of CVD
   C. Modification of risk factors for CVD
      (1) cessation of smoking
      (2) control of hypertension
      (3) control of bone metabolism
      (4) fluid control
      (5) treatment of anemia
      (6) healthy weight control
   D. Therapeutic lifestyle changes (TLC)
      (1) diet and weight management
      (2) increased physical activity
      (3) moderation in alcohol consumption
2. Teach and reinforce self-management skills and strategies
3. Teach patient to report onset of changes in symptoms

Teach and reinforce self-management skills and strategies

Advanced Practice Nursing Care

(In addition to items outlined above)

Assessment

1. Assess the patient for coronary heart disease (CHD) risk equivalent conditions
   A. Clinical CHD
   B. Coronary artery disease (CAD)
   C. Peripheral arterial disease (PAD)
   D. Abdominal aortic aneurysm (AAA)
   E. Diabetes mellitus (DM)
2. Assess patient for modifiable risk factors for CVD and initiate a treatment plan for risk factor reduction

Dyslipidemia – Cardiovascular

3. Interpret results of laboratory tests
4. Monitor patient's response to the treatment plan
   A. CVD risk factor reduction
   B. Therapeutic life changes
   C. Diet prescription
   D. Medication regimen
5. Monitor patient's ability to follow the treatment plan

Intervention

1. Order diagnostic studies and monitor frequency of laboratory testing
2. Adjust medication regimen as appropriate, based on patient response
3. Adjust diet prescription based on assessment of patient

References

Expert Panel on Detection, Evaluation and Treatment of High Blood Cholesterol in Adults (ATP III Guidelines). (2003). Executive summary of the third report of the National Cholesterol Education Program (NCEP) Expert Panel On Detection, Evaluation, and Treatment of High Blood Cholesterol in Adults (Adult Treatment Panel III). *Journal of the American Medical Association, 285*, 2486-2497.

National Kidney Foundation. (2003b). KDOQI clinical practice guidelines for managing dyslipidemias in chronic kidney disease. *American Journal of Kidney Diseases, 41*(4)(Suppl. 3), S1-S91.

Electrolyte Balance

Patient Outcome

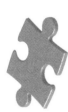

The patient will achieve and maintain electrolyte balance.

The patient will be free of complications related to electrolyte imbalance.

Nursing Care

Assessment

1. Assess changes from previous results
   A. Sodium
   B. Potassium
   C. Calcium
   D. Chloride
   E. Magnesium
2. Assess for dysrhythmias associated with serum elecrolyte imbalance
3. Assess electrolyte intake from all sources
4. Assess fluid status as it relates to serum sodium and albumin levels
5. Assess patient's condition for factors contributing to electrolyte imbalance
6. Assess for correct dialysate and dialysate additives

Intervention

1. Collaborate with physician or advanced practice nurse for adjustments in medications and dialysate composiition as needed based on patient assessment and laboratory results
2. Obtain and review laboratory tests as ordered or according to established protocols
3. Obtain 12-lead electrocardiogram (EKG), if indicated, to interpret cardiac disturbances

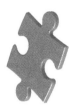

Family Process

Patient Outcome

The patient's family will demonstrate effective coping strategies.

Nursing Care

Assessment

1. Assess past and current coping methods, communication patterns, interactions, roles, and resources
2. Assess interactions and relationships between patient and family
3. Assess family's comprehension of patient's diagnosis and treatment
4. Assess impact of patient's disease and treatment on the patient's family, including physical, social, economic, emotional, and psychological
5. Identify and describe the impact of any behaviors demonstrated by the family that impact the patient's care

Intervention

1. Provide a supportive and accessible environment for the family and patient to discuss feelings and perceptions
2. Encourage and teach the patient's family to become involved in and informed about patient's treatment and care
3. Assist patient and family to identify actual or potential behaviors that may hinder adherence to prescribed treatment
4. Provide positive reinforcement for effective use of coping mechanisms
5. Collaborate with the health care team, including the patient and family, to facilitate communication and problem solving
6. Assist support family/system to identify the need for and use of resources
7. Request social service consultation as needed

Patient and Family Teaching

Before teaching begins, consider health literacy and individualize the approach by considering patient's and family's cultural and health beliefs, preferences, and wishes

1. Review the effects of chronic kidney disease (CKD) and requirements of kidney replacement therapy to include impact on mental health
2. Teach skills that enhance self-management
3. Teach and reinforce communication and problem-solving techniques
4. Describe the stages of adaptation to chronic illness
5. Discuss the emotional impact of the disease process and chronic illness
6. Review stages of expected childhood development and current level of patient functioning for pediatric patients
7. Reinforce the purpose of, and need for, advance care planning and directives
8. Clarify the purpose and availability of end-of-life care

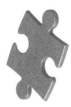

Fluid Balance and Congestive Heart Failure

Patient Outcomes

The patient will be euvolemic and normotensive.

The patient will be on minimal antihypertensive medications.

The patient will not develop congestive heart failure (CHF).

The patient will not be hospitalized for fluid related issues.

The patient will maintain residual kidney function.

The patient will demonstrate knowledge of the implications of optimal fluid balance.

Nursing Care

Assessment

Assess patient for symptoms and root cause of hypervolemia vs. hypovolemia

1. Assess the patient's
   A. Weight: estimated dry weight compared to predialysis and postdialysis weight
   B. Degree of ultrafiltration and ultrafiltration rate (UFR) related to weight, age, comorbidities that may affect fluid status and removal
   C. Blood volume monitor (BVM) profile type, slope, and degree of plasma refill at end of treatment if available
   D. Temperature and changes between predialysis and postdialysis
   E. Blood pressure (lying, sitting, and standing) predialysis, intradialysis, postdialysis
   F. Dose, type, timing, and continued need for BP medications
   G. Heart rate and sounds: apical and peripheral pulses (quality, rate, rhythm)
   H. Respiratory rate and quality, breath sounds, and oxygen needs
   I. Neck vein distention, jugular venous pressure
   J. Capillary refill
   K. Edema: peripheral, facial, periorbital
   L. Skin turgor and mucous membranes
   M. Condition and patency of vascular access
   N. Mental status changes and general sense of well-being
   O. Ability to walk, gait changes
   P. Intake: oral, parenteral, tube feedings
   Q. Output including fluid losses related to residual urine output, draining wounds, nasogastric tube, fever, diarrhea, ileostomy, diaphoresis, hyperventilation, and ultrafiltration
   R. Extravasation of fluids related to bowel dysfunction, ascites, and lymphocele
   S. Changes in abdominal girth measurement
   T. Amount of urine output per 24 hours
   U. Response to and continued need for diuretics
   V. Diet and fluid allowance prescription and adherence
   W. Appetite quality, variation in appetite, and degree of thirst
   X. Sodium intake: source and amount
   Y. Medication: types, doses, regimens, and adherence
   Z. Dialysate type and composition

**Fluid Balance –
Congestive
Heart Failure**

2. Assess patient for symptoms and root cause of hypervolemia vs. hypovolemia
   A. Interdialytic symptoms
      (1) hypertension
      (2) orthostatic hypotension, light-headedness, dizziness
      (3) weakness, fatigue
      (4) muscle cramping
      (5) respiratory difficulties: shortness of breath, dyspnea on exertion, orthopnea
      (6) GI symptoms: nausea, vomiting, diarrhea, changes in appetite
      (7) edema
      (8) thirst level, changes
      (9) decreases in urinary output
      (10) reported recovery time posttreatment
   B. Intradialytic symptoms
      (1) hypertension
      (2) hypotension
      (3) tachycardia, arrhythmia
      (4) chest pain
      (5) nausea, vomiting
      (6) dizziness, changes in sensorium or vision
      (7) muscle cramping
3. Review laboratory test results
   A. Blood urea nitrogen (BUN) and serum creatinine
   B. Electrolytes: calcium, magnesium, potassium
   C. Hemoglobin and hematocrit
   D. Albumin
   E. Atrial and brain natriuretic peptides
   F. Acid-base balance/serum Co_2 level
   G. Serum sodium
   H. Serum glucose/glycosylated hemoglobin
   I. Carnitine level
   J. Angiotension level
   K. Residual kidney function
   L. Cardiac enzymes
4. Review results of diagnostic studies
   A. Electrocardiogram (EKG)
   B. Chest x-rays
   C. Echocardiogram
   D. Blood volume monitor (BVM) profile, type, slope, and degree of plasma refill if available
   E. Sleep studies if ordered
5. Assess the patient's understanding of fluid management and its relationship to congestive heart failure if appropriate

**Assess the
patient's
understanding
of fluid
management**

Intervention

1. Collaborate with physician and dietitian in determining appropriate sodium and fluid intake allowances
2. Review medication regimen for possible causes of symptoms and potential changes
3. Provide instructions and parameters for which and when medications are to be held predialysis and resumed posttreatment
4. Maintain a dialysis log summarizing relevant information that provides a longitudinal dynamic view of extracellular volume and blood pressure changes such as body weight, blood pressure, intradialytic symptoms, and when available, BVM profile and degree of plasma refill

**Fluid Balance –
Congestive Heart
Failure**

5. Review dialysis prescription with interdisciplinary team to determine appropriate, individualized, UF goal, related patient medical history, dialysis time, dialysate composition, temperature, and pH to promote optimal fluid management
6. Monitor patient's response to above prescription and adjust as needed
7. Administer oxygen to prevent symptoms or treat hypoxemia and/or sleep apnea
8. Blood volume monitoring in children < 35 kg
9. Reevaluate medical justification for and avoid or eliminate intradialytic administration of sodium (oral, parenteral, and/or in dialysate) whenever possible
10. Reevaluate residual urine output at least quarterly and adjust or discontinue diuretics as appropriate
11. Administer and monitor fluids according to prescribed treatment plan
12. Encourage adherence to prescribed sodium, fluid, and dietary regimens
13. Encourage adherence to medication regimen
14. Identify resources to assist patient to achieve fluid management goals
15. Identify root causes of symptoms
16. Initiate or request consultations as appropriate

Patient Teaching

Before teaching begins, consider health literacy and individualize the approach by considering patient's cultural and health beliefs, preferences, and wishes

**Instruct patient
regarding
kidney function
and its
relationship to
fluid balance**

1. Instruct patient regarding
   A. Kidney function and its relationship to fluid balance
   B. Adequacy of delivered dialysis dose and its relationship to fluid balance
   C. Blood pressure and its relationship to fluid balance
   D. Prevention and management of hypertension and CHF as related to the patient's current sodium, fluid intake, and medications
   E. The three compartmental fluid shifts occurring during dialysis (extracellular, intracellular, and intravascular) in relation to attaining dry weight and preventing symptoms
   F. Relationship of fluid management to anemia status, albumin level, vascular access flow
   G. Signs, symptoms, and potential causes of hypervolemia and hypovolemia
   H. Signs and symptoms that may occur not related to volume status
   I. Causes, signs, symptoms, and long-term-effects of cardiac alterations related to fluid excess or deficit
   J. Diet and fluid prescription
      (1) daily allowance in relationship to urinary output
      (2) qualification of "fluid" food sources
      (3) recommended weight gains between treatments and relationship to fluid
      (4) recommended UFR for age, weight, prescribed time, and comorbidities
   K. Sodium allowance and sources: dietary and intradialytic
   L. Thirst management and relationship of sodium and glucose
   M. Reading and comprehension of food labels related to sodium content
   N. Effects of eating during the dialysis treatment on fluid management
   O. Relationship of dialysis time and UFR to achieve dry weight
   P. Effects of daily exercise to assist with fluid management
   Q. Triggers and stressors that affect fluid management and techniques to deal with them
   R. Knowledge of when to take or hold BP medications before and after dialysis
   S. Home monitoring
      (1) when and how to weigh self and take BP measurement

Fluid Balance – Congestive Heart Failure

(2) specify parameters to be reported to the nurse

T. For patients receiving peritoneal dialysis, review appropriate use of various dextrose concentrations and monitoring of daily ultrafiltration from dialysis treatment

Advanced Practice Nursing Care

(In addition to items outlined above)

Assessment

1. Interpret results of diagnostic studies (e.g., laboratory tests, EKG, chest x-ray, echocardiogram, sleep studies, residual kidney function, BVM profile, type, slope, and degree of plasma refill, bioimpedance spectroscopy [BIS] if available)
2. Review fluid management effects on anemia, serum albumin, and vascular access patency
3. Monitor patient's adherence to treatment plan
4. Monitor patient's response to treatment plan
5. Review hospitalization admitting diagnosis for accuracy in identifying those related to inaccurate fluid management
6. Analyze dialysis log summarizing longitudinal dynamic view of extracellular volume and blood pressure changes
7. Analyze the root cause of intradialytic morbidities

Intervention

Review fluid management effects on anemia, serum albumin, and vascular access

1. Treat fluid balance, CHF, and hypertension following the most current KDOQI clinical practice guidelines
   A. Lifestyle modifications: counsel on sodium and fluid allowances
   B. Blood pressure target <130/80 mmHg or as ordered by the physician
   C. Adjust medication regimen as appropriate based on patient response
      (1) Adjust or discontinue antihypertensive agents as indicated
      (2) Diuretic adjustments as indicated if urinary output is >100mL/qd
   D. Wean off or avoid sodium profiling
2. Order diagnostic studies as appropriate (e.g., laboratory tests, EKG, chest x-ray, echocardiogram, sleep studies, residual kidney function, BVM type, slope, and plasma refill checks)
3. Adjust sodium, fluid, and dietary prescriptions based on assessment of patient's response to treatment
4. Modify dialysis prescription as needed: time, frequency, ultrafiltration, dialysate composition, and temperature
5. Reevaluate target dry weight as needed
6. Order longer or extra treatment if medically justified to attain dry weight

References

Centers for Medicare & Medicaid Services. (2008) *Conditions for coverage for end stage renal disease facilities: Final rule, Federal Register.* Retrieved from http://www.cms.gov/cfcsandcops/downloads/esrdfinalrule0415.pdf

Mitchell, S. (2002). Estimated dry weight (EDW): Aiming for accuracy. *Nephrology Nursing Journal,* 29(5), 421-428.

National Kidney Foundation. (2006b). NKF-KDOQI clinical practice guidelines on blood pressure management and use of antihypertensive agents in chronic kidney disease. *American Journal Kidney Diseases, 48*(1)(Suppl. 1), S1-183.

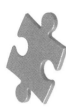

Integrity of Skin and Mucous Membranes

Patient Outcome

The patient will maintain skin and mucous membranes that are clean, intact, and free of infection, pruritus, ecchymoses, subcutaneous calcification, and altered sensation.

Nursing Care

Assessment

1. Assess skin for changes in color, temperature, turgor, texture, vascularity, and sensation
2. Inspect skin for pruritic rash, ecchymoses, purpura, signs of infection, and changes in moles
3. Evaluate patient's skin care practices including sun exposure and use of protective creams and lotions
4. Inspect mouth, gums, and teeth for redness, swelling, bleeding, lesions, thrush, and in patients taking cyclosporine, for gingival hyperplasia
5. Evaluate patient's ability to relieve pressure on bony prominences
6. Review serum chemistries for effectiveness of diet and medication regimens
7. Monitor adequacy of replacement therapy
8. Assess for acne in the posttransplant patient

Intervention

1. Apply creams and ointments and administer prescribed medications for relief of itching, infections, and acne
2. Encourage patient to avoid dehydration and overhydration
3. Encourage 15–30 minutes sun exposure daily for vitamin D creation and the use of sunscreen for longer exposure
4. Administer treatments as prescribed
5. Reinforce adherence to phosphate-binding medications as ordered
6. Assure prescription for antibiotic prophylaxis for invasive dental procedures
7. Encourage patient to regularly change position on weight-bearing prominences if indicated

Patient and Family Teaching

Before teaching begins, consider health literacy and individualize the approach by considering patient's and family's cultural and health beliefs, preferences, and wishes

1. Discuss skin alterations related to uremia
2. Teach therapeutic skin care practices
3. Teach patient self-care measures for skin problems
4. Teach how to identify overhydration and dehydration
5. Teach how to assess and report changes in skin integrity
6. Teach how to assess and report sensory changes
7. Discuss skin alterations related to transplant medications
8. Teach the importance of regular dental care and of informing dentist of chronic kidney disease, dialysis, or transplant status
9. For bladder-drained pancreas recipients, teach methods to avoid perianal excoriation from urinary amylase

Discuss skin alterations related to transplant medications

Integrity of Skin and Mucous Membranes

Advanced Practice Nursing Care

(As outlined above, plus the following)

Assessment

1. Assess patient's response to the treatment regimen

Intervention

1. Prescribe antipruritic medications, antibiotics, or topical creams as indicated

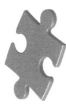

Nutrition and Metabolic Control

Patient Outcome

The patient will achieve and maintain a healthy body weight, good nutritional status, and metabolic balance.

Nursing Care

Assessment

Obtain dietary consultation and ensure regular follow-up by a renal dietitian

1. Assess patient's knowledge and understanding of nutritional requirements
2. Assess pre-illness dietary habits and cultural or ethnic values regarding food preferences, eating patterns, and personal appearance
3. Assess for pica behavior and/or eating disorders (bulimia, anorexia)
4. Assess nutritional status
   A. Weight and body mass index (BMI)
   B. Biochemical data
       (1) blood urea nitrogen
       (2) potassium
       (3) protein, albumin, prealbumin
       (4) calcium
       (5) phosphorus
       (6) hemoglobin, hematocrit
       (7) total lymphocyte count as indicated
       (8) glucose, glycosylated hemoglobin
       (9) lipid studies
       (10) magnesium
       (11) serum bicarbonate
       (12) sodium
       (13) cyclosporine or tacrolimus levels if appropriate
   C. Normalized protein catabolic rate (nPCR)
   D. Clinical appearance and pertinent health history
   E. Anthropometric measurements and/or subjective global assessment (SGA)
   F. Gastrointestinal conditions affecting appetite, nausea, and ability to absorb nutrients
   G. Presence and condition of teeth and condition of gums
   H. Food allergies
   I. Meal planning and meal patterns
5. Assess psychosocial factors that contribute to adherence to prescribed diet and medication regimen

Nutrition and Metabolic Control

6. Assess adequacy of dialysis treatment regimen
7. Assess patient's self-reported sense of well-being
8. Assess for steroid use

Intervention

1. Assist patient to identify a healthy weight
2. Assist patient to integrate the diet as appropriate
3. Administer nutritional supplements as prescribed
4. Encourage adequate dietary intake
5. Obtain dietary consultation and ensure regular follow-up by a renal dietitian
6. Refer to social services as needed to assure availability of appropriate food, supplements, and medication

Patient Teaching

Before teaching begins, consider health literacy and individualize the approach by considering patient's cultural and health beliefs, preferences, and wishes

1. Discuss with patient the importance of dietary modifications and medication therapy, including
   A. Nutritional requirements
      (1) energy
      (2) protein
      (3) sodium and fluid
      (4) potassium
      (5) vitamins
      (6) calcium and phosphorus
      (7) other minerals
   B. Diet prescription
      (1) foods allowed within diet prescription and based on patient's preferences
      (2) foods to be limited
      (3) foods and salt substitutes to avoid
      (4) fluid restriction
      (5) nutritional supplements
   C. Medications, including over-the-counter supplements, antacids, and laxatives
   D. Drug, food, and herbal interactions
2. Teach, reinforce, and assist patient regarding
   A. How to incorporate the prescribed diet to satisfy food preferences and lifestyle
   B. Preparation and use of nutritional supplements as appropriate
   C. How a healthy weight is determined
   D. How to monitor blood glucose, signs and symptoms of hyperglycemia and hypoglycemia, and how to administer glucose-regulating medications
   E. How to read food labels for specific content
   F. Importance of exercise including increased bone density with weight-bearing exercise
   G. Potential for weight gain following transplantation and the importance of maintaining reasonable body weight
   H. Impact of obesity
   I. Importance of regular dental care and of informing dentist and hygienist of chronic kidney disease, dialysis, or transplant status

Discuss with patient the importance of dietary modifications and medication therapy

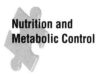

Nutrition and Metabolic Control

Advanced Practice Nursing Care
(In addition to items outlined above)

Assessment
1. Assess patient's response to current prescribed diet

Intervention
1. Collaborate with other health care team members as needed
2. Order nutritional supplements as needed
3. Reinforce patient teaching
4. Collaborate with the health care team regarding referral for gastric bypass in the morbidly obese patient

References

National Kidney Foundation. (2000b). K/DOQI clinical practice guidelines for nutrition in chronic renal failure. *American Journal of Kidney Diseases, 35*(6)(Suppl. 2), S1-S140. Erratum in: (2001). American Journal of Kidney Diseases, 38(4), 917.

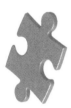

Rehabilitation

Rehabilitation is defined as the process by which patients, family, and support system members work with professionals to achieve the outcomes of optimal physical, social, emotional, psychological, and role functioning in the presence of a potentially disabling condition.

Patient Outcomes

Patient and health care team will mutually agree that despite the constraints imposed by kidney disease, the patient is maximizing functioning or has a plan in place to maximize functioning in four key domains
1. Physical functioning
2. Role functioning (social)
3. Mental health functioning (emotional, psychological)
4. Overall health-related quality of life (QOL) and life satisfaction

Nursing Care

Assessment
1. Physical functioning
    A. Assess patient's ability to perform physical activities required for preferred lifestyle
    B. Explore patient's understanding of exercise requirements for healthy living
    C. Assess level of patient's current regular exercise performance
    D. For pediatric patients, assess whether physical abilities are developmentally appropriate for age
    E. Determine patient's physiologic abilities and limitations
    F. Identify comorbidities that may affect patient's level of activity and ability to exercise (e.g., pain, cardiovascular disease, neuropathies, amputations)
    G. Identify clinical indicators that may affect patient's level of activity and ability to exercise (e.g., residual renal function, adequacy of dialysis, anemia, serum albumin)
    H. Identify deficits in physical functioning (e.g., shortness of breath, hypotension) that may be affected by activity or exercise

Rehabilitation

2. Role functioning
   A. Assess patient's engagement in regular required activities of daily living, including routine and health-related self-care activities
   B. Assess patient's perceptions of ability to perform usual roles and responsibilities in family, larger community, and social circle
   C. Assess patient's ability to participate as fully as desired in preferred social and recreational activities
   D. Assess patient's current employment status and productive activities, including desire to continue or return to work, school, and volunteer activities
   E. Assess patient's level of understanding of the social worker's role as a resource and primary contact for interests, concerns, or problems with employment, job training, school, and volunteer efforts
   F. Determine if patient would benefit from and be interested in consulting with a vocational rehabilitation counselor

3. Mental health functioning
   A. Assess patient's overall psychological status, mood state, and cognitive function
   B. Assess patient's perceptions of and knowledge about diagnosis, prognosis, treatment options, and progress
   C. Identify patient's learning style and any barriers to learning
   D. Assess patient's perception of the role of family members or significant others in caring for and supporting him/her
   E. Consider screening patients for depression with a valid, reliable, depression screening tool (e.g., the Center for Epidemiologic Studies–Depression [CES-D] or Beck Depression Inventory). Though no frequency of screening is recommended in the literature, depression can be present even in the absence of symptoms noted by care team members (see also *Coping* earlier in this section.)

Evaluate patient's ability to set goals and implement, assess, and modify activities

4. Health-related quality of life and life satisfaction
   A. Explore patient's satisfaction with
      (1) health within the constraints of the disease and current treatment modality
      (2) quality of life
      (3) medical care and treatment
   B. Evaluate patient's ability to set goals and implement, assess, and modify activities
   C. Investigate patient's knowledge of and attitude toward self-management, including self-care activities, partnership in care, cooperative decision making, following the treatment regimen, negotiated goals of care and treatment, self-cannulation, and home dialysis
   D. Assess patient's overall attitudes and intentions regarding taking responsibility for aspects of care he/she can control to improve health-related quality of life
   E. Use the KDQOL-36 instrument annually and as needed to quantitate and document patient's perceived QOL for integration into care planning

Intervention

1. Physical functioning
   A. Reinforce the fact that lack of exercise causes loss of muscle tissue and energy
   B. Referral to physical therapy or exercise program as indicated
   C. Collaborate with patient and appropriate members of the health care team to develop an individualized exercise program that is safe and takes into account patient's abilities, health constraints, and motivation
   D. Monitor fitness status (performance measures such as sit-to-stand test) and physical functioning (e.g., SF-36, KDQOL) on a regular basis to track progress and prevent unchecked debilitation

Rehabilitation

    E. Monitor overall activity level (e.g., Disability Interview Schedule) regularly to track potential negative changes in functional status as related to specific activities of daily living

    F. Ensure patient awareness of potential for transplant, home therapies, as well as in-center nocturnal hemodialysis modalities, and their potential benefits and risks

2. Role functioning

    A. Encourage patient to continue to attend and participate in school, work, or volunteer-related activities as much as possible to maintain self-esteem and standard of living

    B. Refer patient to the social worker for employment interests or vocational rehabilitation referral for job skills training and volunteer opportunities

    C. Encourage patient to maintain usual and normal role responsibilities in family and social life and support him/her in their maintenance

    D. Use an activities of daily living (ADL) checklist to identify potential problem areas with regard to role functioning in daily life

    E. Collaborate with patient to identify solutions to role-functioning problems suggested by ADL checklist

    F. Ensure patient awareness of all available modalities

3. Mental health functioning

    A. Monitor overall mental health status, including psychological status, mood state, memory, and cognitive function

    B. Provide information regarding diagnosis, prognosis, and treatment options, and support, guide, and comfort patient as information is assimilated

Empower patient to take responsibility for being a partner in his/her own care

    C. Empower patient to take responsibility for being a partner in his/her own care

    D. Encourage patient to communicate with the health care team by asking questions and sharing important information such as prescription changes and physical symptoms

    E. Encourage patient to tell others what he/she needs and ask for help when needed

    F. Promote patient's sharing of successes with other patients and the health care team and talking with other patients to learn from their experiences

    G. Facilitate the inclusion of patient's family in care decisions and planning to the degree that such family involvement is desired by the patient

    H. Provide an appropriate environment for learning and educational materials that match the patient's learning ability and style

    I. Suggest that patients identified

       (1) discuss depression with the social worker, a clergy person, or other counselor

       (2) ask the nephrologist about antidepressant medications appropriate for use on dialysis

    J. Ensure patient awareness of all modalities available

4. Health-related quality of life and life satisfaction

    A. Encourage and assist patient in setting goals for health care as well as for personal everyday life

    B. Support patient's efforts to maintain independence and to maintain a sense of normality in everyday life

    C. Facilitate family involvement in planning, care, and support to the degree determined by patient

    D. Encourage patient to work toward maximum level of functioning as appropriate for age and condition

    E. Review patient's progress and negotiate a revised plan of action as needed (i.e., plan of care)

Rehabilitation

F. Acquaint patient with principles of self-management for persons with chronic disease, including elements of self-care, partnership in care, cooperative decision making, and negotiated goals of care and treatment

G. Inform patient of the benefits of self-management in terms of functional status, health-related quality of life, and health outcomes

H. Refer patient to other disciplines as appropriate for needs outside the nephrology nursing scope of practice

I. Support and guide patient in the identification of shortcomings or areas of concern with perceived quality of life and with medical care and treatment. Coordinate the formulation of a plan of action to address these issues

J. Ensure patient awareness of transplant, home and in-center hemodialysis modalities, and potential benefits and risks of each

Patient Teaching

Before teaching begins, consider health literacy and individualize the approach by considering patient's and family's cultural and health beliefs, preferences, and wishes

1. Physical functioning: the patient will be taught the following
   A. Lack of exercise causes loss of muscle tissue and energy
   B. Individuals with kidney disease are particularly prone to physical debilitation
   C. Exercise benefits
      (1) decreased stress, anxiety, and depression
      (2) improved self-esteem and feelings of control
      (3) more energy and stronger muscles
      (4) improved control of blood pressure, diabetes mellitus, and cholesterol
      (5) reduced fall risk, less cramping, and increased bone strength
   D. Clinical indicators that may affect patient's level of activity
   E. Begin with simple physical activities that preserve or increase functional ability (e.g., "If you can walk even one step today, you can walk two steps tomorrow, and you can increase that number by a step a day....")
   F. How to monitor overall activity level to track potential negative changes in functional status as related to specific activities of daily living

Include family members as a resource and source of support

2. Role functioning
   A. Value of maintaining work, school, or volunteer-related activities
   B. Importance of maintaining usual and normal role responsibilities in family and social life
   C. Importance of self-monitoring ability to perform regular activities of daily living; use an ADL checklist to identify potential problem areas and to address them as soon as they are identified
   D. How to collaborate with health care team to identify solutions to problems suggested by ADL checklist

3. Mental health functioning
   A. Methods for effectively communicating to the health care team needs, symptoms, and preferences with regard to treatment and health care
   B. Methods to access the health care team as a source of information, support, and guidance
   C. How to share successes with other patients and the health care team
   D. Methods for communicating with the health care team regarding feelings, problems, disappointments, and issues
   E. How to include family members as a resource and source of support
   F. How to attend to own mental health status including mood state, memory, and cognitive function

Rehabilitation

      G. How to take responsibility for partnership in own care

      H. How to report symptoms of depression

  4. Health-related quality of life and life satisfaction

      A. Benefits of rehabilitation

      B. Benefits of following the prescription for treatment, medication, exercise, and nutrition therapy

      C. Kidney disease and how treatments can lessen symptoms and promote healthy living and longevity

      D. Principles of self-management

        (1) integrating treatment into lifestyle

        (2) partnering in care

        (3) communicating with the health care team

        (4) performing self-care activities

        (5) adhering to the treatment regimen

        (6) achieving self-care and self-efficacy

      E. Value of cooperative decision making and negotiated goals of care and treatment

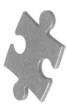

Residual Kidney Function

Patient Outcome

The patient will achieve a urine elimination pattern within physiologic limitations.

The patient will retain as much residual kidney function as possible for as long as possible.

Nursing Care

Assessment

1. Assess patient's current voiding pattern including frequency, quantity of urine, presence of pain with urination, incontinence, or bladder distention

2. Determine patient's previous voiding pattern, history of urologic, nephrologic, or developmental problems including neurogenic voiding difficulties; review medications, especially any affecting ability to void

3. Assess function of urinary diversion system, if applicable

4. Establish baseline information

    A. Intake and output

    B. Weight

    C. Vital signs

    D. Glomerular filtration rate (GFR)

      (1) measured by 24-hour urine collection for creatinine clearance

      (2) estimated by equation

    E. Urinalysis if indicated

    F. Ultrasound or x-ray reports

5. Assess for abnormalities of urine, including pyuria, hematuria, stones, and foul odor

6. Assess for changes in volume of urine output and voiding pattern

7. Check for postvoid residual when indicated

8. Assess presence and degree of proteinuria

Residual Kidney Function

Intervention

1. Encourage patient adherence to prescribed fluid and medication regimens
2. Encourage patient to report changes in voiding pattern, frequency, and quantity of urine output
3. Encourage patient to report presence and degree of fluid retention
4. Encourage patient to express concerns arising from urologic problems
5. Catheterize bladder as appropriate
6. Preservation of residual kidney function
   A. Avoid nephrotoxic drugs
      (1) intravenous radiocontrast agents
         a. if unavoidable, selected low or iso-osmolar nonionic contrast agents in limited amounts decreases risk
         b. gadolinium should not be used for imaging in individuals with glomerular filtration rates below 30 mL/min due to the risk of nephrogenic systemic fibrosis
      (2) aminoglycosides
      (3) nonsteroidal antiinflammatory drugs
   B. Avoid dehydration
   C. Protective measures if intravenous contrast is unavoidable
      (1) IV hydration prior to the procedure
      (2) discontinue diuretics, renin-angiotensin-aldosterone blocking agents 24 hours prior to procedure
      (3) administer protective medications prior to the procedure (current recommendation is for acetylcysteine 1200 mg PO every 12 hours on the day prior to and the day of the contrast procedure, isotonic IV sodium bicarbonate solution)
      (4) control of blood pressure
   D. Control proteinuria

Patient Teaching

Before teaching begins, consider health literacy and individualize the approach by considering patient's cultural and health beliefs, preferences, and wishes

1. Discuss with patient
   A. Physiologic changes caused by kidney disease
   B. Goals of fluid and medication regimens
   C. How to measure intake and output
   D. Signs and symptoms to report to health care team
2. Reinforce need to maintain personal cleanliness and appropriate skin care
3. Educate patient regarding
   A. Diagnostic testing used to evaluate the urinary tract system
   B. Techniques required for urinary self-catheterization or diversion as appropriate
   C. How to measure blood pressure emphasizing individual blood pressure goal

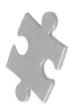

Sexuality – Adult

Patient Outcome

The patient will feel sexual issues have been addressed as needed.

The patient will maintain his/her desired level of sexuality and sexual activity.

Nursing Care

Assessment

1. Assess current level of knowledge and beliefs regarding impact of disease and treatment regimen on sexuality and sexual function
2. Assess patient's fears and anxieties related to sexual functioning
3. Determine if patient is taking medications that affect sexual functioning (e.g., antihypertensives, antidepressants, antihistamines)
4. Assess risk for sexually transmitted diseases
5. Identify sexual function goals

Intervention

1. Explore causative and contributing factors for dysfunction if applicable
2. Discuss meaning of sexuality and previous sexual history with patient and significant other
3. Explore how change in sexual function impacts masculine/feminine role
4. Encourage communication between patient and significant other
5. Initiate or request referrals as needed
6. Encourage patient to talk with prescriber (or the interdisciplinary team member he/she is most comfortable talking to) about medications that impact sexual function
7. Educate patient to never stop or skip medications, but to take them as prescribed
8. Encourage safe sex practices

Patient Teaching

Before teaching begins, consider health literacy and individualize the approach by considering patient's cultural and health beliefs, preferences, and wishes

1. Dispel myths and misconceptions about sex and kidney disease and provide information on normal sexuality, sexual issues with kidney disease, and treatment options for sexual dysfunction as needed
2. Provide information/instruction about alternative methods of achieving sexual satisfaction and ways of treating sexual dysfunction when patient and significant other are receptive to learning
3. Emphasize the importance of giving and receiving love and affection
4. Discuss changes in sexual activity after initiation of replacement therapy or transplantation
5. Discuss birth control with the sexually active patient
6. Discuss measures to prevent transmission of, or exposure to, sexually transmitted diseases
7. Discuss measures to prevent urinary tract infections, especially posttransplant
8. Discuss the possibility of pregnancy with the sexually active patient, and with the posttransplant patient

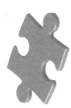

Sexuality – Adolescent

Patient Outcome

The patient will experience age-appropriate sexual development.

Nursing Care

Assessment

1. Assess patient's and parents' current level of knowledge of impact of disease on sexual development
2. Assess patient's and parents' concerns about adolescent's sexual development
3. Determine current sexual activity
4. Assess sexual development using Tanner staging: http://www.brightfutures.org/georgetown.html
5. Assess status of vaccines (i.e., human papillomavirus [HPV])

Intervention

1. Encourage the patient to verbalize concerns, anxieties, and fears to the health care team and parents
2. Initiate or request referrals as needed
3. Assist patient in achieving goals with sexuality

Patient Teaching

Before teaching begins, consider health literacy and individualize the approach by considering patient's cultural and health beliefs, preferences, and wishes

1. Discuss expected changes in sexuality after initiation of replacement therapy
2. If sexually active, discuss potential for disinterest in, decreased capability for, or discomfort during sexual activity; discuss strategies to overcome these barriers
3. Discuss possibility of pregnancy and birth control measures with the sexually active patient
4. Discuss measures to prevent exposure to and transmission of sexually transmitted diseases
5. Discuss measures to prevent urinary tract infections, especially posttransplant
6. Provide information on sexual function or sexuality as needed to patient and family

References

Georgetown University. Bright futures. Retrieved from http://www.brightfutures.org/georgetown.html
Tanner, J.M. (1962). *Growth at adolescence* (2nd ed.). Oxford, England: Blackwell Scientific Publications.

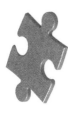

Self-Concept and Self-Management

Patient Outcomes

The patient will become an active, comprehensive self-manager of his/her life with chronic disease. Specifically, the patient will

- Integrate treatment regimen into his/her preferred lifestyle.
- Communicate regularly and effectively with members of health care team.
- Partner in care, participate in decision-making, and collaborate in the development of plan of care.
- Request, obtain, and understand health-related information.
- Follow treatment regimen that has been negotiated with health care team members.
- Perform appropriate self-care activities as determined in cooperation with the health care team members including home dialysis treatments and self-cannulation of a vascular access if possible.
- Exhibit self-care self-efficacy, defined as confidence in ability to effectively perform self-care activities and produce the desired outcomes.

Nursing Care

Assessment

Assess the patient's
1. Primary language: reading comprehension level and ability to communicate verbally
2. Previous and current lifestyle, role expectations, and role performance
3. Previous and current support systems in family and social networks
4. Religious, spiritual, and cultural beliefs
5. Educational background and occupational, professional, and personal goals
6. Response to the impact of illness on family, financial status, and the patient's ability to manage cost of treatment and lifestyle changes
7. Previous health experiences and culturally specific resources used including orientation to, and experience with, the health care system
8. Barriers to health care and lifestyle adaptations
9. Past experience with, as well as expectations for, a working relationship with the health care team
10. Perception of and knowledge about disease, treatment, progress, and prognosis
11. Need and desire for specific information about the disease and its treatment, and optimal role in own care
12. Past experiences with and effectiveness of self-care
13. Current level of self-management
14. Suitability for transfer to in-center self-care or for home treatment: peritoneal dialysis or home hemodialysis (conventional, short daily, or nocturnal)
15. Ability to overcome any barriers identified to home treatment

Intervention

1. Establish pattern of partner-oriented communication with patient in which patient's input is solicited for health care decisions
2. Partner with the patient to develop a plan of care that supports the patient's level of readiness, positive coping skills, and self-management abilities

Self-Concept and Self-Management

3. Discuss and negotiate alternative patient behaviors that are congruent with changes in personal relationships, lifestyle, and role performance
4. Discuss potential resources and refer patient to support groups, patient organizations, and online resources appropriate for topics in which patient expresses interest
5. Encourage patient to verbalize concerns about changes in body image, lifestyle, close relationships, role expectations, and life goals
6. Consult with patient about self-management
    A. Acquaint patient with the concept of comprehensive self-management as outlined in the outcomes listed above
    B. Acknowledge patient's current self-management practices
    C. Negotiate ongoing self-management goals and activities
7. Determine the patient's level of confidence in his/her ability to accomplish specific self-management goals
8. Consult with health care team members regarding the need for outside service referrals as indicated
9. Identify and determine how to overcome barriers to transplant, home dialysis, or self-care treatment

Patient Teaching

Before teaching begins, consider health literacy and individualize the approach by considering patient's cultural and health beliefs, preferences, and wishes

Determine the patient's level of confidence in his/her ability to accomplish specific self-management goals

1. Provide appropriate information about the disease, its treatment, progress, and prognosis based on the patient's expressed interest, ability to comprehend, and readiness to self-manage
2. Provide information on the impact of each ESRD treatment modality on lifestyle factors important to the patient, including
    A. Diet
    B. Fluid limits
    C. Medications
    D. Ability to work, travel, and sleep
    E. Sexuality and fertility
    F. Symptoms
    G. Hospital stays
    H. Survival
3. Provide information that describes self-management and verifies its success in terms of patient satisfaction as well as health outcomes
4. Provide information regarding the specific expectations of both patients and health care team members in a patient self-management relationship
5. Instruct patient about the processes involved in active participation in care planning and self-management goal setting
6. Provide anticipatory guidance and counseling that address major stressors and barriers to change
7. Provide opportunity for patient to meet others who have had similar experiences
8. Provide the opportunity for a peer partner who can encourage and assist patient in successful self-management

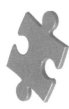

Sleep

Patient Outcomes

The patient will achieve and maintain restorative sleep.

The patient will achieve and maintain optimal daytime alertness.

Nursing Care

Assessment

Chief complaint is usually expressed as insomnia, excessive daytime sleepiness, or unwanted nocturnal behaviors, movements, or sensations

1. Assess general sleep habits, regularity, and duration of sleep
   A. Time it takes to fall asleep
   B. Average number of hours obtained nightly
   C. Perceived quality of sleep
   D. Typical time to go to bed and arise (if on hemodialysis, review for both dialysis and nondialysis days)
   E. Recent changes in sleep patterns, including before and after the initiation of dialysis
   F. Presence of bed partner and his/her perception of the patient's sleep
   G. Exercise habits, especially immediately prior to bedtime
   H. Duration and timing of light exposure
   I. Stress levels
   J. Habitual patterns of food, caffeine, and alcohol ingestion
   K. Anxiety, depression
   L. Medications, including those taken for sleep promotion (prescribed and over-the-counter)
2. Assess for insomnia
   A. Difficulty falling asleep, staying asleep, or early morning awakenings
   B. Factors that may prevent patient from falling or staying asleep
   C. Sleep environment: noise, light, distractions, interruptions
   D. Awakenings during the night
   E. Average number of awakenings, reason for awakenings, and how long it takes to fall back to sleep
3. Assess for excessive daytime sleepiness
   A. Levels of daytime sleepiness, including unintentional sleep episodes
   B. Likelihood of falling asleep when reading, watching TV, during a conversation, while driving
   C. Difficulty concentrating
   D. Social or work-related problems
4. Assess for unwanted nocturnal behaviors, movements, or sensations
   A. Behaviors, movements, sensations that may disturb sleep such as itching, pain, leg cramps, diaphoresis, dyspnea, breath holding, gasping, or gastroesophageal reflux
   B. Snoring
   C. Witnessed apnea
   D. Kicking or twitching of legs or arms at night
   E. Irresistible urge to move or other types of sensations in the arms or legs that become worse in the evening and are relieved by movements (e.g., restless legs [RLS])
   F. Dreams or nightmares

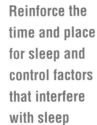

Reinforce the time and place for sleep and control factors that interfere with sleep

Table 4.1

Selected Instruments Available for the Assessment and Measurement of Nocturnal Sleep and Daytime Sleepiness

Nocturnal Sleep

Instrument	Description	Reference
Leeds Sleep Evaluation Questionnaire	10-item visual analogue scale often used to assess response to sleep medications Measures sleep latency (time it takes to fall asleep), sleep quality, and daytime alertness	Parrott, A. C., & Hindmarch, I. (1980). The Leed's Sleep Evaluation Questionnaire in psychopharmacological investigations – A review. *Psychopharmacology, 71*, 173-179.
Pittsburgh Sleep Quality Index	24-item fill-in-the-blank instrument Has section for bed partner ratings in addition to self-rated parameters Measures sleep quality, sleep latency, sleep duration, sleep efficiency (time asleep/time in bed x 100), sleep disturbance, use of sleeping medication, and daytime dysfunction	Buysse, D. J., Reynolds, C. F., Monk, T. H., Berman, S. R., & Kupfer, D. J. (1989). The Pittsburgh Sleep Quality Index: A new instrument for psychiatric practice and research. *Psychiatry Research, 28*(2), 193-213.
The St. Mary's Hospital Sleep Questionnaire	14-item fill-in-the-blank instrument Designed for use with inpatients Measures sleep quality, sleep latency, sleep duration, sleep disturbance, and daytime alertness	Ellis, B. W., Johns, M. W., Lancaster, R., Raptopoulos, P., Angelopoulos, N., & Priest, R. G. (1981). The St. Mary's Hospital Sleep Questionnaire: A study of reliability. *Sleep, 4*(1), 93-97.
National Sleep Foundation Sleep Diary	Fill-in-the-blank record of sleep patterns Table format allows for comparison of multiple days on one page Measures sleep quality and daily practices that affect sleep (activity, naps, caffeine, etc.)	National Sleep Foundation. (1999). National Sleep Foundation Sleep Diary. Available: http://www.sleepfoundation.org
Pittsburgh Sleep Diary	Fill-in-the-blank record of sleep patterns and visual analogue scales Measures sleep quality and daily practices that affect sleep (activity, naps, caffeine, etc.)	Monk, T. H., Reynolds, C. F., Kupfer, D. J., Buysse, D., Coble, P. A., Hayes, A. J., Machen, M. A., Petrie, S. R., & Ritenour, A. M. (1994). The Pittsburgh Sleep Diary. *Journal of Sleep Research, 3*, 111-120.

Daytime Sleepiness

Instrument	Description	Reference
Stanford Sleepiness Scale	Seven items (one is selected) related to level of alertness/sleepiness Measures current state of introspective sleepiness	Hoddes, E., Zarcone, V. P., Smythe, H., Phillips, R., & Dement, W. C. (1973). Quantification of sleepiness: A new approach. *Psychophysiology, 10*(4), 431-436.
Epworth Sleepiness Scale	Eight-item scale Measures likelihood of falling asleep in everyday situations	Johns, M. W. (1991). A new method for measuring daytime sleepiness: The Epworth Sleepiness Scale. *Sleep, 14*(6), 540-545.

Sleep

5. Use available tools for the subjective assessment of both nocturnal sleep and daytime sleepiness (see Table 4.1)

Nonpharmacologic Interventions

Nonpharmacologic interventions focus on promoting adequate restful and restorative sleep and optimizing daytime alertness. Reinforce the time and place for sleep and control factors that interfere with sleep

1. General sleep hygiene
   A. Avoid inconsistent and lengthy daytime naps; limit naps to 1 hour per day unless otherwise indicated
   B. Limit the time in bed to the average number of hours actually slept per night; too much time in bed can decrease sleep quality on the subsequent night
   C. Use the bedroom for sex and sleep only; don't bring work or other related activities into the bedroom
   D. Get regular exercise each day; finish exercise 4 to 6 hours before bedtime
   E. Keep a regular sleep/wake schedule
   F. Avoid bright light at night, but get 30 minutes of sunlight early in the day
   G. Avoid smoking, caffeine, and alcohol
   H. Keep the clock face turned away if it becomes upsetting
   I. Keep the room dark, quiet, well ventilated, and at a comfortable temperature
   J. Avoid unfamiliar sleep environments
   K. Setting aside planned "worry time" an hour or two before bedtime may be helpful to decrease anxiety and racing thoughts
   L. Keep in mind that sleep changes with age; sleep is normally less deep with age
2. Relaxation techniques
   A. Produce a calm inner state through reduction of arousal
      (1) Massage may reduce anxiety and induce sleep
      (2) Music therapy may enhance relaxation
      (3) White noise such as ocean, rain, and waterfall sounds may decrease arousal
3. Body position *before* sleeping may have beneficial effect on some patients
   A. Side position or elevating head of the bed may facilitate optimal breathing
      (1) Snoring, gasping, or apneas
   B. Weight loss may be indicated
4. Patient-reported sleep diary
   A. Use when impaired sleep is a significant ongoing problem
   B. Document frequency and severity of symptoms and their effect on daily activities
   C. Evaluate progress of treatment
   D. Promote self-management

Pharmacologic Interventions

1. Use short-acting benzodiazepine-like agents such as zaleplon, zopiclone, or zolpidem (used primarily for acute insomnia)
   A. Can be used safely in dialysis patients
   B. When abruptly discontinued, sleep may worsen (rebound insomnia), an effect that can be reduced by tapering the dose
   C. Patients with sleep apnea or heavy snoring are not good candidates for hypnotic medications as drugs may worsen hypoxemia and the related sleep disturbance
   D. Long-term use of hypnotics has been associated with increased risk of mortality in the general population
2. Analgesics or other medications administered for pain relief when indicated

Explain the role of chronic kidney disease and its impact on sleep

Sleep

3. Administer medications for anxiety and/or depression if these conditions are present
   A. Selected antidepressants and antipsychotics may trigger
      (1) development or worsening of restless legs syndrome (RLS) symptoms
      (2) periodic limb movements
   B. Treatment of low iron saturation and ferritin with iron replacement may decrease restless leg symptoms and periodic limb movements
4. Monitor patient closely for medication side effects

Patient Education

Before teaching begins, consider health literacy and individualize the approach by considering patient's cultural and health beliefs, preferences, and wishes

1. Explain the role of chronic kidney disease and its impact on sleep
2. Discuss the importance of good sleep
3. Explain possible adverse effects of herbal or over-the-counter sleep medications
4. Explain the diagnostic tests used to evaluate sleep disorders (e.g., polysomnography)
5. Teach patient about general behavioral strategies, relaxation techniques, and body postures that promote good sleep
6. Teach patient about any medication prescribed for sleep, including expected results and side effects
7. Request referral to a sleep specialist for the following disorders
   A. Sleep apnea with history of snoring, witnessed apnea, gasping during sleep, daytime sleepiness
   B. Periodic limb movement disorder with symptoms of nocturnal kicking, jerking, daytime sleepiness
   C. Restless legs syndrome characterized by irresistible urges to move legs; becomes worse during rest and at night, and is relieved by movement or standing

Advanced Practice Nursing Care

(As outlined above, plus the following)

Assessment

1. Assess patient for sleep pathology as indicated

Intervention

1. Order and review results of diagnostic studies
2. Prescribe appropriate sleep aids
3. Collaborate with other health care providers as needed

References

American Academy of Sleep Medicine – www.aasmnet.org

National Sleep Foundation – www.sleepfoundation.org

Parker, K.P., Kutner, N.G., Bliwise, D., Bailey, J.L., & Rye, D.B. (2003). Nocturnal sleep, daytime sleepiness, and quality of life in stable patients on hemodialysis. *Health and Quality of Life Outcomes*, 1, 68. doi: 10.1186/1477-7525-1-68. Retrieved from http://www.ncbi.nlm.nih.gov/pmc/articles/PMC320494

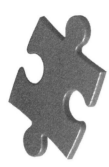

Infection Control

115	**Bacterial Infection**
117	**Hepatitis B**
119	**Hepatitis C**
120	**Tuberculosis**

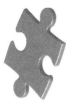

Bacterial Infection

Patient Outcome

The patient will be free of signs and symptoms associated with localized infection or sepsis.

The patient's risk for bacterial colonization or infection due to a drug-resistant organism will be reduced.

Nursing Care

Assessment

1. Identify factors in the patient's environment, lifestyle, health practices, and comorbid conditions (e.g., DM, PVD, and HIV) that may increase the risk of infection
2. Assess patient's personal hygiene practices
3. Assess for signs and symptoms of infection
    A. Hyperthermia, with or without chills
    B. Catheter insertion site, AV graft, AV fistula for local areas of induration, warmth, swelling, tenderness, erythema, and drainage
    C. Hypotension or hemodynamic instability
    D. Tachycardia
    E. Generalized weakness and fatigue
    F. Night sweats
    G. Confusion
4. Monitor laboratory test results, including Gram stain, cultures and sensitivities, white blood cell count and differential, and indicators of nutritional status (e.g., albumin, total protein)

Intervention

1. Obtain laboratory analyses and cultures as ordered
    A. Obtain cultures prior to starting antibiotic therapy
        (1) Blood cultures
            a. Use proper antisepsis for drawing blood cultures
            b. Obtain one peripheral vein blood culture, if possible, per order
            c. Avoid culturing vascular catheter tips, surrounding skin, or catheter hub
            d. Requisition special tests as ordered (e.g., cultures for anaerobes or fungi)
        (2) Catheter exit site or wound cultures
            a. culture exudate when present

Bacterial Infection

    B. Notify the physician or advanced practice nurse of culture results
       (1) Report initial Gram stain results as soon as possible
       (2) Report final culture and sensitivity results, noting the presence of a drug-resistant organism as soon as possible
    C. Obtain repeat culture per order
2. Collaborate with physician and advanced practice nurse to avoid overuse of vancomycin
3. Administer antibiotics and other medications as prescribed
4. Monitor patient response (e.g., resolution of infection, development of sepsis)
5. Perform dressing changes according to established protocol
6. Provide nursing care according to unit infection control policies and procedures that are consistent with the Centers for Disease Control and Prevention (CDC) guidelines (2001; 2002) and current NKF KDOQI Vascular Access Guidelines
7. Strict adherence to infection control practices as recommended for all dialysis patients
8. Consider additional precautions for treatment of patients who might be at increased risk for transmitting pathogenic bacteria (e.g., patients with an infected skin wound with drainage that is not contained by dressings, fecal incontinence, or diarrhea uncontrolled)
9. Additional precautions may include wearing a separate gown, removing the gown when finished caring for the patient, and dialyzing the patient at a station with as few adjacent stations as possible (e.g., at the end or corner of the unit)
10. Assist patient to alter personal health habits as appropriate

Patient Teaching

Teach patient signs and symptoms of infection to report to nurse

Before teaching begins, consider health literacy and individualize the approach by considering patient's cultural and health beliefs, preferences, and wishes

1. Teach patient basic principles of infection control
2. Discuss manifestations of uremia as they relate to potential for infection
    A. Immune system suppression
    B. Potential for bacterial colonization and infection of access
    C. Importance of permanent vascular access placement rather than long-term use of a hemodialysis catheter
    D. When to replace dressing (e.g., catheter has sufficient drainage to dampen or soil the dressing)
3. Reinforce importance of adherence to prescribed nutrition, medication, and fluid regimens
4. Teach patient signs and symptoms of infection to report to nurse
5. Discuss or reinforce good hygiene practices
    A. Hand washing
    B. Care of the vascular access
    C. Washing the vascular access prior to dialysis
    D. Glove use when holding vascular access site to stop bleeding
    E. Peritoneal catheter exit site care
6. Reinforce the importance of home dialysis patients performing procedures as instructed
7. Discuss immunosuppressive medication as it relates to potential for infection
8. Discuss use of prophylactic antibiotic therapy for the patient with a transplant or new PD catheter as appropriate
9. Teach the patient the importance of informing nephrology team of any antibiotics ordered by other health care providers
10. Discuss the importance of immunizations as recommended by the CDC, including the annual seasonal influenza vaccine

Bacterial Infection

11. Teach importance of good skin care (e.g., foot checks for patients with diabetes, pressure points in patients with limited mobility)

Advanced Practice Nursing Care

(In addition to items outlined above)

Assessment

1. Assess patient risk factors for infection

Intervention

1. Order and interpret diagnostic tests (e.g., blood culture, urine culture, complete blood count, chest x-ray, indicators of nutritional status, antibiotic levels)
2. Order antibiotics as indicated
3. Monitor patient response to treatment regimen
4. Refer as appropriate to other health care providers

References

Campaign to Prevent Antimicrobial Resistance in Dialysis Patients. Centers for Disease Control and Prevention. http://www.cdc.gov/drugresistance/healthcare/patients.htm#dialysis

Centers for Disease Control and Prevention (1995). Recommendations for preventing the spread of vancomycin resistance recommendations of the Hospital Infection Control Practices Advisory Committee (HICPAC). *Morbidity and Mortality Weekly Report, 44*(RR-12).

Centers for Disease Control and Prevention (2001). Recommendations for preventing transmission of infections among chronic hemodialysis patients. *Morbidity and Mortality Weekly Report, 50*(RR-5).

Centers for Disease Control and Prevention (2002). Guidelines for the prevention of intravascular catheter-related infections. *Morbidity and Mortality Weekly Report, 51*(RR-10).

National Kidney Foundation. (2006d). NKF-KDOQI clinical practice guidelines for vascular access: Update 2006. *American Journal of Kidney Diseases, 48*(1)(Suppl. 1), S176-S307.

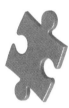

Hepatitis B

Patient Outcomes

The patient will not convert to HBsAg-positive status.

Hepatitis B will not be transmitted in the dialysis unit.

Liver damage secondary to hepatitis B will be minimized.

Nursing Care

Assessment

1. Hepatitis B virus (HBV) surveillance as recommended by the Centers for Disease Control and Prevention (CDC)
   A. Hepatitis B surface antigen (HBsAg), antibody to hepatitis B surface antigen (anti-HBs), and hepatitis B total core antibody (anti-HBc) for all new patients prior to admission
   B. HBsAg monthly for all HBV-susceptible patients including nonresponders to the hepatitis B vaccine, those who have not yet received the vaccine, and those who are in the process of receiving the vaccine

Hepatitis B

C. Anti-HBs annually for all anti-HBs positive (>10 mIU/mL) patients who are hepatitis B total core antibody (anti-HBc) negative, indicating vaccine-induced immunity

2. Assess for signs and symptoms of hepatitis
    A. Jaundice
    B. Anorexia
    C. Nausea and vomiting
    D. Arthralgia
    E. Fever
    F. Abdominal pain

3. Elicit history of exposure to hepatitis

Intervention

1. Provide HBV vaccine according to physician or advanced practice nurse orders and facility policy, consistent with the CDC guidelines
    A. Vaccinate all susceptible patients
    B. Test for anti-HBs 1–2 months after last dose of vaccine series
    C. If anti-HBs is ≥10 mIU/mL, consider the patient immune, retest annually and provide a booster dose of vaccine if <10 mIU/mL
    D. If anti-HBs is <10 mIU/mL, consider the patient susceptible, revaccinate with a second full series, and retest for anti-HBs 1–2 months after last dose of the second vaccine series
    E. Consider patient a vaccine non responder if anti-HBs <10 mIU/mL and continue to test monthly for the hepatitis B surface antigen (HBsAg)

2. Provide nursing care according to unit infection control policies and procedures that are consistent with the CDC guidelines
    A. Dialyze HBsAg-positive patients in a separate room, using separate machines and supplies
    B. HBsAg-positive patients must not participate in dialyzer reprocessing program
    C. Staff members caring for HBsAg-positive patients should not care for HBV-susceptible patients at the same time

3. Minimize use of anticoagulants in the patient with liver disease if platelets are depleted

4. Administer monotherapy with alpha interferon or lamivudine, adjusted for creatinine clearance, per physician order and facility medication administration policy, for the HBsAg-positive patient

5. Collaborate with physician and advanced practice nurse to adjust medications with potential hepatotoxicity, including immunosuppressant drugs and acetaminophen-containing analgesics

6. Assess the patient with chronic liver disease for immunization with the hepatitis A vaccine to prevent additional liver damage

Patient Teaching

Before teaching begins, consider health literacy and individualize the approach by considering patient's cultural and health beliefs, preferences, and wishes

1. Explain rationale for hepatitis B surveillance and modes of transmission
2. Teach infection control practices appropriate for unit and home
3. Provide information regarding hepatitis immunization
4. Instruct patient regarding potential side effects associated with alpha interferon therapy
5. Provide examples of appropriate over-the-counter pain medications and those to avoid

Vaccinate all susceptible patients

Hepatitis B

6. Instruct patient to notify health care team of new medications, either prescribed or over-the-counter
7. Discuss potential treatment options and interventions for HBsAg-positive patients

Advanced Practice Nursing Care

(In addition to items outlined above)

Assessment

1. Medication toxicity
2. Abnormal liver enzymes, clotting factors
3. Hepatitis B immunization history
4. Presence of antibodies

Intervention

1. Adjust medications as needed
2. Order hepatitis B vaccine if indicated
3. Refer to specialist as needed

NOTE

HBsAg positive test results: The Department of Health and/or other appropriate agencies will be notified according to state protocol.

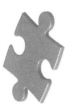

Hepatitis C

Patient Outcomes

The patient will not convert to a positive anti-HCV status.

The patient with a positive anti-HCV will not transmit the disease.

Liver damage will be minimized in the patient with hepatitis C virus (HCV).

Nursing Care

Assessment

1. Monitor hepatitis C surveillance laboratory test results
   A. Antibody to hepatitis C virus (anti-HCV) and alanine aminotransferase (ALT) on admission for all patients
   B. ALT monthly for anti-HCV negative patients
   C. Anti-HCV for all negative anti-HCV patients per accepted recommendations and guidelines
   D. Supplemental testing with more specific assays (e.g., RIBA, HCV RNA nucleic acid testing) for patients with an initial positive anti-HCV requiring confirmatory testing
2. Assess for persistently abnormal or unexplained elevated ALT levels
3. Elicit history of exposure to hepatitis

Intervention

1. Provide nursing care according to unit infection control policies and procedures that are consistent with the Centers for Disease Control and Prevention (CDC) guidelines
   A. Strict adherence to infection control practices as recommended for all hemodialysis patients

Hepatitis C

B. Isolation is not recommended

C. Dialyzing on a dedicated machine is not recommended

2. Minimize use of anticoagulants in the patient with liver disease if platelets are depleted

3. Collaborate with physician and advanced practice nurse to adjust medications with potential hepatotoxicity, including immunosuppressants and acetaminophen-containing analgesics

4. Assess the patient with chronic liver disease for immunization with the hepatitis A vaccine to prevent additional liver damage

Patient Teaching

Before teaching begins, consider health literacy and individualize the approach by considering patient's cultural and health beliefs, preferences, and wishes

1. Explain rationale for hepatitis C surveillance and the modes of transmission

2. Teach the patient how to prevent further liver damage

3. Teach the patient how to prevent hepatitis C transmission to others

4. Explain appropriate use of over-the-counter medications

5. Instruct patient to notify health care team of new medications, either prescribed or over-the-counter

6. Explain the importance of following through with prescribed referrals for evaluation and treatment of chronic liver disease

NOTE

Anti-HCV positive test results: The Department of Health and/or other appropriate agencies will be notified according to state protocol.

Reference

Centers for Disease Control and Prevention. (2003). Guidelines for laboratory testing and result reporting of antibody to hepatitis C. *Morbidity and Mortality Weekly Report, 52*(RR03), 1-16.

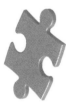

Tuberculosis

Patient Outcomes

The patient will not convert from a negative to a positive tuberculosis (TB) skin test.

The patient will not progress to active TB disease.

The patient with active TB will not transmit the disease.

Nursing Care

Assessment

1. Monitor laboratory test results related to TB screening, diagnosis, and treatment
   A. Mantoux skin test
   B. Chest x-ray
   C. Sputum smear and culture
   D. Quantiferon-TB Gold (QFT-G)

2. Assess for signs and symptoms of TB (e.g., symptom screen or risk appraisal)
   A. Productive or persistent cough
   B. Cloudy or blood-tinged sputum
   C. Unexplained weight loss

Tuberculosis

    D. Night sweats
3. Elicit history of exposure to TB
    A. Living with a person who has active TB
    B. Recent travel to locations where TB is common
    C. Exposure to possibly infected persons
    D. Live or work in crowded conditions (e.g., prisons, nursing homes, homeless shelters)
    E. Poor access to health care prior to chronic kidney disease (CKD) or dialysis (e.g., migrant worker, homeless)
4. Assess for risk factors that increase the risk of development of active TB disease after exposure
    A. Immunosuppression
    B. Human immunodeficiency virus (HIV)
    C. History of TB or positive skin test without treatment or completion of prescribed medication
5. Monitor adherence medication regimen for patients receiving therapy for either latent TB infection (LTBI) or active TB disease

Intervention

1. Provide TB screening per current recommendations of the Centers for Disease Control and Prevention (CDC) and physician or advanced practice nurse order
2. Provide nursing care according to unit infection control policies and procedures that are consistent with current CDC guidelines
3. Patients with active contagious TB of the lung, airways, or larynx must be cared for in a health care facility that provides for isolation in an airborne infection isolation (AII) room
4. Administer medications as prescribed
5. Coordinate care with other health care providers and agencies as indicated (e.g., local health department)

Patient Teaching

Before teaching begins, consider health literacy and individualize the approach by considering patient's cultural and health beliefs, preferences, and wishes

1. Explain rationale for TB surveillance
2. Teach respiratory infection control practices
3. Reinforce importance of adherence to prescribed medication regimen
4. Teach patient signs and symptoms of disease progression to report to nurse

NOTE

TB skin test conversions and active cases of TB disease: The Department of Health and/or other appropriate agencies will be notified according to state protocol.

References

Centers for Disease Control and Prevention. (2001). Recommendations for preventing transmission of infections among chronic hemodialysis patients. *Morbidity and Mortality Weekly Report, 50*(RR-5).

Centers for Disease Control and Prevention. (2005a). Guidelines for preventing the transmission of *Mycobacterium tuberculosis* in health-care settings. *Morbidity and Mortality Weekly Report, 54*(RR-17).

Centers for Disease Control and Prevention. (2005b). Guidelines for the investigation of contacts of persons with infectious tuberculosis: Recommendations from the National Tuberculosis Controllers Association and the CDC. *Morbidity and Mortality Weekly Report, 54*(RR-15).

Centers for Disease Control and Prevention. (2010). Updated guidelines for using interferon gamma

Tuberculosis

release assays to detect *Mycobacterium tuberculosis* infection. *Morbidity and Mortality Weekly Report, 59(RR-5)*.

Siegel, J., Rhinehart, E., Jackson, M., Chiarello, L., & the Healthcare Infection Control Practices Advisory Committee, Centers for Disease Control and Prevention. (2007). Guideline for isolation precautions: Preventing transmission of infectious agents in healthcare settings. Retrieved from http://www.cdc.gov/hicpac/2007IP/2007isolationPrecautions.html

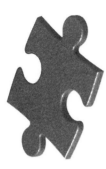

Hemodialysis

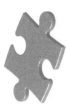

Vascular Access

Patient Outcomes

The patient's vascular access will provide a blood flow rate adequate to achieve the dialysis prescription.

The patient's vascular access will have a long use life and be free of complications.

The patient and patient's family will demonstrate knowledge regarding his/her vascular access.

Nursing Process

Assessment

1. General observations
   A. Fluid status
   B. Vital signs (including pain observation)
   C. Self-management: able to wash access, protect from injury
   D. Affect
   E. Subjective data
      (1) Assess self-report of any abnormal signs or symptoms or medical interventions since previous dialysis treatment at facility
      (2) Assess patient's subjective response to the vascular access (e.g., body image, self-concept, fears)
2. Assess the patient's access extremity for
   A. Type of access (AVF, AVG, AVG hybrid, or buttonhole)
   B. Location and integrity of incisions
   C. Pulses
   D. Swelling
   E. Presence of collateral veins
   F. Change in color or temperature
   G. Areas of numbness or decreased sensation
   H. Limitations of movement
   I. Change in both gross and fine motor function
   J. Capillary refill in nailbeds >2 seconds
   K. Comparison to contralateral extremity

Vascular Access

3. Focused assessment of AVF or AVG. Absence of
   A. Redness
   B. Ecchymosis
   C. Hematoma
   D. Rash or break in skin
   E. Drainage from previous cannulation sites including buttonholes
   F. Bleeding
   G. Warmth or coolness of digits
   H. Tenderness or pain
   I. Aneurysm or pseudoaneurysm
   J. Stenosis: ascertain vein collapse (partial or full) of AVF outflow vein when arm raised above head
   K. Cannulation considerations
      (1) maturation of AVF
      (2) maturation and health of buttonholes in AVF if appropriate
      (3) incorporation of AVG
      (4) direction of blood flow identified and documented
      (5) auscultate for bruit from arterial anastomosis throughout the cannulation area of the access
      (6) palpate arterial, mid, and venous sections of cannulation area for presence, absence, and character of pulse or thrill
      (7) plan for rotation of cannulation sites in AVG, AVG hybrid, and AVF; assess for the potential for creation of buttonholes in AVF
      (8) choose both needle sites prior to cannulation and intended direction of the arterial needle
      (9) assess intended location of needle tip, staying away from anastomoses by at least the length of the needle
      (10) appropriate gauge and length of needle

Solicit access complaints from patient and evaluate prior to initiation of treatment

4. Assessment related to the dialysis catheter prior to dialysis
   A. Verify catheter tip position before first use, if not placed under fluoroscopy
   B. Verify absence of
      (1) any respiratory distress
      (2) cardiac arrhythmia
      (3) facial or neck edema
   C. Check catheter for integrity of catheter caps, hubs, tail, and dressing
   D. Look for a well-healed exit site, with absence of
      (1) redness
      (2) induration or swelling
      (3) discoloration or bruising
      (4) drainage or bleeding
      (5) evidence of catheter migration (visible cuff if using cuffed catheter)

5. Solicit access complaints from patient and evaluate prior to initiation of treatment
   A. Access problems during or since the last treatment
   B. Pain or tenderness at the access or exit site
   C. Sensations of coldness, numbness, tingling, or pain in access extremity
   D. Impairment of movement in access limb
   E. Bleeding or drainage from cannulation site or exit site
   F. Fever or chills

6. Assess the patient during the treatment for
   A. Degree of pain during cannulation and effectiveness of preventive measures

Vascular Access

B. Sequellae of difficult cannulation
   (1) pain
   (2) infiltration or hematoma
C. Needles taped securely
D. Connections: visible and secure
E. Difficulty achieving or maintaining prescribed blood flow rate
F. Assess for mechanical or thrombotic dysfunction in catheters (if BFR is < 300 mL/min)
G. Arterial or venous pressure outside the established parameters
H. Bleeding or oozing from cannulation site or catheter exit site
I. Pain
J. Temperature greater than established parameter
K. Air/foam in lines

7. Assess AVF or AVG for hemodynamically significant stenosis using one of the following
   A. Intra-access flow measured monthly (AVF or AVG, AVG hybrid)
   B. Static venous dialysis pressure every 2 weeks (AVG and AVG hybrid)
   C. Computer-derived static pressures
   D. Dynamic venous pressure monitoring and urea-based recirculation measurements are no longer recommended by the KDOQI guidelines for access surveillance

Interventions

1. Notify the physician or advanced practice nurse of any assessment findings that require alteration in the hemodialysis treatment plan
2. Cannulate AVF or AVG following established current KDOQI guidelines
   A. Wash hands; wear gloves and PPE (personal protective equipment)
   B. If rotating sites, select sites away from previous sites
   C. Use rope ladder technique with AVG; a light tourniquet may be used with AVG for assessment and cannulation if graft difficult to feel
   D. Use rope ladder or same-site buttonhole technique with AVF; always use a tourniquet
   E. Do not cannulate into aneurysms or pseudoaneurysms
   F. Needle tips should be spaced sufficiently to avoid recirculation between needles
      (1) Enough room should be left between needles to compress vessel and assess for recirculation
   G. Clean skin following established policies that are consistent with KDOQI guidelines
   H. Cannulate access and tape needles securely
   I. Connect patient per protocol and check for complications over the first 1–2 minutes
   J. Maintain visibility of the access and connections at all times
3. Catheter connection and disconnection
   A. Wash hands; wear gloves and PPE. Patient must also wear a mask!
   B. Clean catheter hub/connection following established policies that are consistent with CDC guidelines with 2% chlorhexidine or povidone iodine; allow to dry and then separate (povidone-iodine must be dry for 2 minutes)
   C. Minimize the time that the catheter lumens are open to air
   D. Withdraw locking solution minimizing amount of blood removed
   E. Flush each lumen with 10 mL of normal saline to assess catheter patency and integrity; if catheter patency is abnormal, assess for mechanical or thrombotic dysfunction
   F. Institute lytic therapy as per facility protocol if thrombotic dysfunction diagnosed
   G. Connect patient per protocol and check for complications over the first 1–2 minutes

Do not cannulate into aneurysms or pseudoaneurysms

Vascular Accesss

H. Maintain visibility of access and connections at all times

I. Postdialysis, repeat steps A through C

J. Flush each lumen with 10 mL of normal saline to clear lumens of any remaining blood

K. Lock each lumen with solution following unit protocol

L. Assure cap security

M. Change dressing either each treatment or weekly following unit protocol

4. Monitor access function at least every 30 minutes during the treatment

 A. Blood flow rate

 B. Arterial pressure

 C. Venous pressure

5. Postdialysis, remove needles from AVF or AVG

 A. Compress the peripheral sites with two fingers following complete removal of the needle

 B. Do not occlude the blood flow in peripheral access (check pulse distal to the site of pressure)

6. Evaluate findings indicative of stenosis and report to nephrologist and/or advanced practice nurse

 A. Edema of access extremity

 B. Appearance of collateral veins

 C. Outflow vein of AVF not partially collapsed with arm elevation (predialysis)

 D. Postdialysis bleeding time >30 minutes with usual heparin dose

 E. Difficulty with cannulation

 F. Pain

 G. Altered characteristic of thrill or bruit

 H. Recent pseudoaneurysm formation in AVG

7. Treat AVF or AVG complications

 A. Infiltration: intermittent use of ice for the first 24 hours, then warm compresses

 B. Bleeding: attempt hemostasis; if bleeding persists, report to nephrologist, advanced practice nurse, or vascular surgeon

 C. Poor flow: reposition needles; treat hypovolemic hypotension if present

 D. Infection: do not cannulate; obtain culture, report findings, and initiate antibiotic therapy as ordered

8. Report to vascular access team (specifically nephrologist, advanced practice nurse, or surgeon)

 A. Poor healing of cannulation sites and any thinning or break in skin covering aneurysms or pseudoaneurysms

 B. Thrombosis

 C. Ischemia in limb

 D. Any sign of infection

 E. Prolonged bleeding

 F. Abnormal results of AVF or AVG monitoring

 G. Complications with catheter

9. Treat catheter complications

 A. Poor flow: thrombolytic agent per order if not a mechanical problem

 B. Infection: obtain culture, report findings, and initiate antibiotic therapy as ordered

 C. Bleeding from new exit site: attempt hemostasis with gauze dressing; if bleeding persists, report to nephrologist or advanced practice nurse

10. Initiate consultations or request referrals as appropriate

> **Maintain visibility of access and connections at all times**

Vascular Access

Patient and Family Teaching

Before teaching begins, consider health literacy and individualize the approach by considering patient's and family's cultural and health beliefs, preferences, and wishes

1. Instruct patient and family/support system regarding
   A. Purpose and type of access
   B. Preferred access type generally and specifically for the patient
   C. Care and protection of access and future access sites
   D. How to assess for patency of AVF or AVG
   E. Signs and symptoms of infection and information to report to nurse
   F. Signs and symptoms of complications, management strategies, and information to report to nurse
   G. Rotation of cannulation sites or care of buttonholes as appropriate
   H. Proper cannulation techniques (with avoidance of aneurysms or pseudoaneurysms)
   I. Proper compression of access for hemostasis
   J. Emergency care
   K. Benefits of self-cannulation if suitable
   L. Assist patient in identifying activity and clothing appropriate for vascular access type and site

Advanced Practice Nursing Care

(In addition to items outlined above)

Maintain a plan for future access if current access fails

Assessment

1. Monitor the patient's overall vascular access function
2. Review dialysis adequacy laboratory results
3. Assess the patient's vascular access for complications, including hemodynamic compromise
4. Assess the patient's peripheral vascular system and cardiovascular system for future access sites

Interventions

1. Collaborate with the nephrologist to formulate a plan for optimal hemodialysis access
2. Maintain a plan for future access if current access fails
3. Educate patient about vein preservation for future access creation
4. Evaluate patient for complications related to the vascular access
5. Order laboratory tests and diagnostic studies as appropriate
6. Initiate evaluation and treatment of peripheral access complications
   A. Inadequate flow
   B. Hemodynamically significant venous stenosis
   C. Thrombosis
   D. Infection
   E. Vein or graft degeneration and aneurysm/pseudoaneurysm formation with
      (1) risk of rupture
      (2) evidence of spontaneous bleeding
      (3) compromised skin overlying aneurysm/pseudoaneurysm
      (4) limited available cannulation sites
   F. Ischemia (steal syndrome) in limb with or without pain
   G. Loss of or change in normal function
   H. Unacceptable body image

Vascular Access

NOTE
Pediatric patients: Per the KDOQI guidelines of 2006, the blood flow rate of an external access should be minimally 3–5 mL/kg/min and should be adequate to deliver the prescribed HD dose.

References

Centers for Disease Control and Prevention (CDC). (2002). Guidelines for the prevention of intravascular catheter-related infections. *Morbidity and Mortality Weekly Report, Recommendations and Reports, 51*(RR-10A), 1-29

Dinwiddie, L.C. (2008). Vascular access for hemodialysis. In C. Counts (Ed.), *Core curriculum for nephrology nursing* (5th ed., pp. 735-764). Pitman, NJ: American Nephrology Nurses' Association.

National Kidney Foundation. (2006d). KDOQI clinical practice guidelines for vascular access: Update 2006. *American Journal of Kidney Diseases, 48*(1)(Suppl. 1), S176-S307.

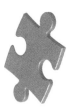

Adequacy

Patient Outcomes

The patient will have a delivered dose of hemodialysis that meets or exceeds the KDOQI and CMS Conditions of Coverage target for adequate dialysis.

The patient will demonstrate knowledge of the hemodialysis prescription and the importance of the delivered dose of dialysis.

The patient will demonstrate adherence to the hemodialysis prescription.

The patient's level of functioning will be maintained or improved.

The patient will describe a satisfactory quality of life.

Nursing Care

Assessment

1. Measure the delivered dose of hemodialysis at least monthly, using urea kinetic modeling (Kt/V), and compare to recommended KDOQI target Kt/V
   A. Kt/V single-pool urea kinetic modeling is preferred and most precise
   B. Urea reduction ratio (URR) is acceptable
   C. Conductivity (ionic) clearance underestimates dialyzer urea clearance
2. Measure residual kidney function at least quarterly
3. Assess patient for signs and symptoms of inadequate dialysis
   A. Abnormal electrolytes
   B. Hypervolemia
   C. Hypertension/numerous antihypertensive medications
   D. Left ventricular hypertrophy
   E. Symptoms of uremia
   F. Worsening nutritional status
   G. Anemia
   H. Bone disease
   I. Neuropathies
   J. Abnormal sleep patterns, insomnia
   K. Neurologic symptoms (e.g., restless legs, difficulty concentrating)

Adequacy

L. Poor quality of life

M. Abnormal growth and development in children

N. Poor vocational or school performance

O. Prolonged recovery time postdialysis

4. If the actual delivered dose of hemodialysis falls below the target level, assess potential reasons

  A. Compromised urea clearances

    (1) inadequate access blood flow

    (2) access recirculation

    (3) inappropriate dialyzer size or clearance

    (4) inadequate dialyzer reprocessing

    (5) excessive dialyzer clotting during dialysis

    (6) inadequate extracorporeal blood flow rate

    (7) inadequate dialysate flow rate

    (8) dialyzer leaks

    (9) incorrect prime technique: introduction of air in dialyzer

    (10) incorrect needle placement or reversal of blood lines

  B. Reduction in treatment times

    (1) inaccurate assessment of effective treatment time (e.g., use of wall clock or watch instead of machine treatment time)

    (2) uncompensated interruptions in actual treatment time

      a. occurrence of clinical complications such as hypotension/cramping during treatment

      b. equipment alarms

      c. manipulation of needles

      d. dialysate bypass situations (e.g., temperature or conductivity alarms)

    (3) shortened treatment time

      a. premature discontinuation of dialysis due to

        [1] patient request or demand

        [2] dialysis unit issues, such as facility hours, patient schedule restraints, limited staff availability

        [3] clinical complications

      b. delay in initiation of dialysis

        [1] patient issues: late for treatment, access problems

      c. missed dialysis treatments

  C. Laboratory or blood sampling errors

    (1) sampling methods

    (2) timing of sampling

    (3) laboratory error

5. Assess the patient for causes of intradialytic complications that could potentially result in inadequate delivered dose of dialysis

  A. Inaccurate estimated dry weight (EDW)

  B. Large interdialytic weight gains

  C. High ultrafiltration rate

  D. Medication related

  E. Hypoxemia

  F. Anemia

  G. Cardiovascular issues such as poor ejection fraction, arrhythmia, ischemia

  H. Posture

  I. Increased temperature during treatment

  J. Eating during treatment

  K. Inaccurate pre-weight documented

Assess patient's understanding of the importance of the delivered dose of hemodialysis

Adequacy

6. Assess patient's understanding of the importance of the delivered dose of hemodialysis in relationship to long-term effects on morbidity and mortality, and his or her role in achieving adequate dialysis

Intervention

1. Take measures to correct any problems that could potentially result in compromised clearances during dialysis
2. Take measures to correct any problems resulting in reduced dialysis treatment time
3. Initiate measures to identify root causes and decrease intradialytic complications, which could result in a decrease in delivered dose of dialysis
   A. Periodically reassess estimated dry weight (EDW) and results of plasma refill check (if available) with patient's nephrologist or advanced practice nurse
   B. Review patient's dialysis prescription at least monthly with nephrologist or advanced practice nurse
      (1) dialysate sodium concentration needs or removal of sodium profile
      (2) need for use of isolated ultrafiltration
      (3) dialysate temperature
      (4) treatment time and frequency vs. ultrafiltration requirements
      (5) other dialysate constituents (bicarbonate, calcium, glucose, potasssium)
      (6) heparin requirements
4. Ensure that laboratory specimens and data used to determine delivered dose of hemodialysis are collected correctly
   A. Obtain predialysis and postdialysis blood samples for blood urea nitrogen (BUN) at the same dialysis treatment
   B. Obtain blood sample for the predialysis BUN immediately prior to initiation of dialysis using a technique that avoids dilution of the blood sample with saline or heparin
   C. Obtain blood sample for the postdialysis BUN at the end of the prescribed treatment time using a slow flow or stop flow technique
5. Ensure that hemodialyzers are reprocessed following the Association for the Advancement of Medical Instrumentation (AAMI) standards

Ensure that laboratory specimens and data used to determine delivered dose of hemodialysis are collected correctly

Patient Teaching

Before teaching begins, consider health literacy and individualize the approach by considering patient's cultural and health beliefs, preferences, and wishes

1. Discuss the rationale for the recommended dose of hemodialysis and the relationship of the delivered dose to patient outcomes and long-term effects on morbidity and mortality
2. Review elements of the hemodialysis prescription, the importance of adherence to the prescription, and the patient's role in achieving adequate dialysis
3. Explain how dialysis adequacy is measured and the relationship of the patient's size to dialysis time and dialyzer efficiency
4. Review adequacy of dialysis and its relationship to fluid balance
5. Explain the rationale for adherence to dietary, sodium, and fluid recommendations as they relate to achieving adequate dialysis
6. Review patient's medications and explain the importance of adherence to the medication regimen
7. Explain the importance of having a well functioning access to achieve dialysis adequacy

Adequacy

Advanced Practice Nursing Care

(In addition to items outlined above)

Assessment

1. Interpret results of urea kinetic modeling
2. Reassess residual kidney function at least quarterly
3. Monitor prescribed vs. delivered dose of dialysis
4. Monitor patient's response to the hemodialysis prescription
5. Reassess for dry weight changes frequently
6. Analyze results of BVM: profile type, slope, and degree of plasma refill (if available)
7. Clinical assessment for signs of inadequate dialysis
8. Monitor patient's adherence to dialysis prescription
9. Monitor patient's vascular access function
10. Review patient's nutritional status, including normalized protein catabolic rate (nPCR)
11. Assess patient's cardiovascular status
12. Monitor patient's anemia status
13. Monitor for oxygenation needs
14. Reevaluate medications and need for adjustments at least monthly
15. Explore reasons for patient's nonadherence as needed

Intervention

1. Prescribe a hemodialysis dose that will achieve the KDOQI target Kt/V, euvolemia, and normotension
2. Modify the hemodialysis prescription based on patient response to treatment and urea kinetic modeling data
3. Collaborate with interdisciplinary team to identify root causes of intradialytic symptoms and compromising delivered dose
4. Modify the hemodialysis prescription to prevent occurrence of intradialytic symptoms without compromising delivered dose
5. Adjust patient's dry weight based on clinical and BVM assessment (when available)
6. Adjust patient's anemia regimen as appropriate
7. Adjust patient's medication orders based on patient response to treatment
8. Order additional laboratory tests or diagnostic studies as appropriate
9. Initiate consultations or referrals, as indicated

References

Association for the Advancement of Medical Instrumentation – www.aami.org/standards

Centers for Medicare and Medicaid Services. (2008). Conditions for coverage for end stage renal disease facilities: Final rule, Federal Register. Retrieved from http://www.cms.gov/cfcsandcops/downloads/esrdfinalrule0415.pdf

National Kidney Foundation. (2006c). NKF/KDOQI clinical practice guidelines for hemodialysis adequacy. *American Journal of Kidney Diseases, 48*(1)(Suppl 1), S13-97.

Reassess residual kidney function at least quarterly

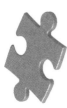

Treatment and Equipment-Related Complications

Patient Outcomes

The patient will receive an appropriate and safe hemodialysis treatment.

The patient will be free of complications of anticoagulation.

The patient will be free of treatment/equipment-induced complications including, but not limited to, hemolysis, pyrogen reaction, dialyzer reaction, air embolism, and exsanguination.

The patient will demonstrate knowledge of the dialysis equipment and procedures and of potential treatment or equipment-related complications.

Nursing Care

Assessment

1. Assess the patient predialysis, intradialysis, and postdialysis
   A. Weight: estimated dry weight compared to predialysis and last postweight
   B. Degree of ultrafiltration/ultrafiltration rate related to dialysis time, patient weight, age, and comorbities that may affect safe fluid removal
   C. Temperature and changes between predialysis and postdialysis
   D. Blood pressure predialysis (sitting, and standing) intradialysis, and postdialysis (sitting, and standing)
   E. Continued need for BP medications and/or dose changes
      (1) Assess if patient held or time BP medications taken pretreatment
   F. Heart rate/sounds: apical and peripheral pulses (quality, rate, rhythm)
   G. Respiratory rate and quality, breath sounds, oxygen needs
   H. Neck vein distention, jugular venous pressure
   I. Capillary refill
   J. Edema: peripheral, facial, periorbital
   K. Skin turgor and mucous membranes
   L. Condition and patency of vascular access
   M. Mental status/changes
   N. General sense of well-being
   O. Reported recovery time posttreatment
   P. Interdialytic symptoms and complaints
   Q. Ability to ambulate, gait changes
   R. Intake: oral, parenteral, and intradialytic fluid intake
   S. Output including all fluid losses; 24-hour residual urine output, draining wounds, nasogastric tube, fever, diarrhea, ileostomy, diaphoresis, hyperventilation, and ultrafiltration
   T. Extravasation of fluids related to bowel dysfunction, ascites, and lymphocele
   U. Changes in abdominal girth measurement
   V. Appetite: changes and degree of thirst
   W. Continuous electrocardiogram (EKG) and pulse oximetry monitoring in children <20 kg; adults as indicated
   X. Blood volume monitoring in children <35 kg; adults as indicated to establish, maintain, and reassess dry weight and assist in prevention and root cause of intradialytic symptoms
   Y. Assess the patient for ecchymoses, hematomas, or other signs of bleeding

Treatment and Equipment-related Complications

    Z. Elicit history of injuries, bleeding, unusual bruising, menses, and surgical procedures

2. Assess the equipment prior to initiation of the prescribed treatment
   A. Equipment suitability and completion of alarm testing
   B. Dialysis machine
      (1) disinfected per facility protocol
      (2) absence of disinfectant
      (3) proper blood pump occlusion
      (4) alarms set and functioning properly
   C. Dialysate
      (1) matches prescription
      (2) appropriate conductivity and pH
      (3) isothermic temperature
   D. Dialyzer
      (1) matches prescription
      (2) check integrity of membrane
      (3) nonreprocessed: follow manufacturer and unit instructions for use
      (4) reprocessed
         a. labeled with correct patient name
         b. presence of sterilant
         c. absence of residual sterilant following rinse
         d. follow unit and Association for the Advancement of Medical Instrumentation (AAMI) standards for reuse
   E. Extracorporeal circuit
      (1) integrity of blood lines
      (2) absence of kinking
      (3) absence of air in dialyzer and blood lines
   F. Treated water
      (1) meets AAMI standards
      (2) absence of disinfectant
      (3) water treatment system alarms function properly

3. Review anticoagulation needs
   A. Regimen type during previous treatments
   B. Previous hemoglobin, hematocrit, calcium, and coagulation studies
   C. Interdialytic changes in condition, signs or risk of bleeding, menses
   D. Recent procedures that have been or are scheduled to be performed
   E. Dialyzer and extracorporeal circuit clotting during and after treatment
   F. Medication history, noting pharmacologic agents affecting anticoagulation, including over-the-counter and nontraditional medicines

4. Monitor the patient throughout the treatment for signs and symptoms of hemolysis
   A. Chest, back or abdominal pain, and possible crescendo of that pain
   B. Dyspnea
   C. Hypotension
   D. Dysrhythmias
   E. Localized burning or pain in access extremity
   F. Clear, translucent deep burgundy, or cherry-red color of blood in venous blood line
   G. Complaint of feeling hot
   H. Acute decrease in Hb/Hct if testing available
   I. Hyperkalemia

5. Monitor the patient throughout the treatment for onset of signs and symptoms of pyrogenic reaction
   A. Temperature elevation within the first 45–75 minutes of dialysis

Assess the equipment prior to initiation of the prescribed treatment

**Treatment and
Equipment-Related
Complications**

    B. Complaint of feeling cold after initiation of dialysis

    C. Chills

    D. Involuntary shaking

    E. Hypotension, hemodynamic instability

    F. Myalgia

    G. Headache

    H. Nausea, vomiting

6. Monitor the patient throughout treatment for onset of signs and symptoms of a membrane bioincompatibility

    A. Type A reaction

        (1) occurs in first 5–10 minutes of treatment

        (2) can progress to anaphylaxis, cardiac arrest, and death

        (3) milder case presents with itching, urticaria, cough, sneeze, watery eyes, or GI symptoms

        (4) signs and symptoms

            a. feeling of uneasiness, warmth, sense of impending doom

            b. agitation

            c. chest tightness

            d. back pain

            e. acute bronchial restriction, dyspnea, respiratory stridor

            f. coughing

            g. wheezing

            h. urticaria

            i. facial edema

            j. flushing

            k. nausea

            l. blood pressure can be high or low

    B. Type B reaction

        (1) Occurs 20–40 minutes after initiation; resolves after first hour

        (2) Signs and symptoms

            a. chest pain

            b. back pain

            c. hypotension

Once dialysis is initiated, assess integrity of the extracorporeal circuit, including connections and delivery system alarms

7. Once dialysis is initiated, assess integrity of the extracorporeal circuit, including connections and delivery system alarms

8. Assess integrity of central venous catheter if present

9. Monitor the patient throughout the treatment for signs and symptoms of air embolism

    A. Visualization of air pockets or foam in venous blood line

    B. Feeling of air rushing into circulation

    C. Sound of a "train" or "rushing air"

    D. Churning sound on auscultation of the heart

    E. Chest pain

    F. Dyspnea, cough

    G. Cyanosis

    H Visual disturbances

    I. Neurologic deficits: confusion, coma, hemiparesis

    J. Cardiac arrest

    K. Death

10. Monitor patient throughout the treatment for signs and symptoms of exsanguination

    A. Obvious bleeding

    B. Hypotension, increased heart rate

    C. Decrease in Hb/HCT if testing available

Treatment and Equipment-related Complications

    D. Shock

    E. Seizures

    F. Cardiovascular collapse, cardiac arrest

11. Assess patient's understanding of the hemodialysis procedure and patient's role in presenting signs and symptoms of potential complications

Intervention

1. Ensure accurate delivery of anticoagulant (intermittent or continuous)
   A. Adjust anticoagulation regimen based on
      (1) coagulation studies
      (2) patient's condition
      (3) patency of extracorporeal circuit and dialyzer
      (4) responses to previous anticoagulation
      (5) postdialysis bleeding of cannulation sites
      (6) recent or scheduled surgical procedures
      (7) increased risk of intracranial hemorrhage in neonates
      (8) physician or advanced practice nurse's order

2. Take appropriate measures to prevent acute hemolysis
   A. Ensure that the extracorporeal system is free of disinfectant prior to initiation of dialysis
   B. Ensure that system alarms are functioning properly
   C. Correct any dialysate conductivity, temperature, or pH problems
   D. Monitor preblood pump arterial pressures to ensure it does not exceed –250mmHg
   E. Use appropriate blood flow rates for type and size of access
   F. Ensure water treatment, distribution, and dialysate preparation meet AAMI standards
   G. Assess extracorporeal system to ensure absence of kinks and other manufacturer defects
   H. Ensure the patient is not left unattended during HD treatment

3. If hemolysis occurs
   A. Stop treatment, clamp all blood lines. Do NOT reinfuse blood
   B. Provide supportive emergency care and oxygen
   C. Notify physician or advanced practice nurse immediately
   D. Obtain blood samples: electrolytes, hemoglobin/hematocrit, bilirubin, haptoglobin, LDH
   E. Monitor BP, heart rate, and rhythm
   F. Replace fluid volume or transfuse as ordered
   G. Collect dialysate samples for analysis
   H. Save extracorporeal circuit for analysis
   I. Attempt to identify root cause of hemolysis
   J. Restart dialysis if ordered, using new equipment and supplies

4. Take appropriate measures to prevent a pyrogenic reaction
   A. Proper water treatment, disinfection of equipment, and reuse procedures per AAMI standards
   B. Proper technique in preparation of dialysate and extracorporeal system
   C. Preparation of extracorporeal system no longer than 2 hours prior to initiation of hemodialysis treatment
   D. Careful preparation of equipment and supplies; aseptic treatment initiation to prevent contamination
   E. Protect patients from infectious agents
   F. Careful handling of bicarbonate concentrate to avoid contamination

Ensure water treatment, distribution, and dialysate preparation meet AAMI Standards

Treatment and Equipment-related Complications

      G. Prevent backflow of dialysate by maintaining minimum UFR

      H. Regular cleaning and disinfection of water treatment and distribution system, dialysate delivery system, and concentrate containers

5. If a pyrogenic reaction occurs

    A. Notify physician or advanced practice nurse

    B. Obtain vital signs, including temperature

    C. Assess for and maintain proper dialysate temperature (34–36 degrees C)

    D. Evaluate other potential sources of infection such as vascular access, foot ulcers, respiratory tract, or urinary tract

    E. Administer antipyretics and antibiotics as ordered

    F. Supportive treatment of symptoms

    G. Discontinue HD without returning blood if a pyrogen or endotoxin reaction is suspected

    H. Obtain cultures

      (1) blood

      (2) treatment water

      (3) dialysate inlet and outlet

    I. Obtain samples of treatment water and dialysate for endotoxin (Limulus amoebocyte lysate [LAL] is the most sensitive test)

6. Take appropriate measures to prevent membrane bioincompatibility

    A. Type A reaction

      (1) if a polyacrylonitrile (PAN) dialyzer is prescribed, review medications to determine if patient is taking an angiotensin-converting enzyme (ACE) inhibitor

      (2) notify physician or advanced practice nurse if patient is taking ACE inhibitor and is prescribed dialysis with a PAN membrane

      (3) ensure that the extracorporeal circuit is properly rinsed prior to initiation of dialysis to remove ethylene oxide sterilant, other sterilants, or allergens

      (4) use of dialyzer sterilized with electron beam, gamma-radiation, or steam to avoid exposure and reactions

      (5) administer antihistamines prior to treatment for patients with milder cases

      (6) change to alternative membrane or sterilant

      (7) place patient in reuse program

      (8) reprocess reuse dialyzers prior to first use

      (9) follow AAMI standards for water treatment

    B. Type B reaction

      (1) change to dialyzer with a more compatible membrane

      (2) monitor throughout treatment for onset of symptoms

      (3) place in reuse program if available

7. If a membrane bioincompatibility occurs

    A. If severe, discontinue dialysis without reinfusing blood (if symptoms resolve with Type B reactions, treatment does not need to be terminated)

    B. Supportive treatment of symptoms

    C. Administer oxygen

    D. Notify physician or advanced practice nurse

    E. Administer intravenous antihistamine, steroids, or epinephrine per order depending on the severity of the reaction

Take appropriate measures to prevent an air embolism

8. Take appropriate measures to prevent an air embolism

    A. Secure all Luer-lok connections and caps on the extracorporeal circuit

    B. Ensure conditions that allow visualization of extracorporeal circuit at all times, including access and connections

Treatment and Equipment-related Complications

    C. Visual inspection of venous blood line before connecting to access

    D. Ensure that air detector is functioning and calibrated

    E. Ensure that any clamps used during the dialysis treatment are occlusive; double clamp saline administration line

    F. Use only non-air-vented bags for intravenous (IV) infusions during treatment

    G. Administer IV fluids as a bolus, rather than as an infusion, unless via an infusion pump

    H. Disconnect or clamp empty IV bags, blood bags, or infusion syringes

    I. Heparin infusion site should be after the blood pump

    J. Maintain blood pump speed at a rate that can be delivered by the access

    K. At termination of dialysis, return blood with saline rinse, not an air rinse

    L. Monitor patient throughout treatment for symptoms; never leave patient unattended

9. If an air embolus occurs
    A. Stop infusion of air immediately and clamp blood lines
    B. Initiate emergency interventions following facility policy that may include
        (1) placing patient in Trendelenberg position and turning on left side
        (2) notifying physician or advanced practice nurse
        (3) administering oxygen (100% by mask is preferred; hyperbaric oxygen therapy may be beneficial if available)
        (4) assessing vital signs and level of consciousness
        (5) monitoring cardiac status (generally cardiac massage should not be attempted until air is removed from right ventricle via needle aspiration)
        (6) supportive treatment of symptoms
    C. Assess and correct possible causes

Ensure conditions that allow visualization of extracorporeal circuit at all times, including access and connections

10. Take appropriate measures to prevent exsanguination
    A. Secure all Luer-lok connections and caps on the extracorporeal circuit
    B. Secure needles with tape
    C. Ensure conditions that allow visualization of extracorporeal circuit at all times, including access and connections
    D. Ensure properly functioning blood detector and pressure alarms
    E. Appropriately cap and secure central venous catheters
    F. Place blood lines properly in blood pump
    G. Connect both arterial and venous blood lines to access lines at initiation of HD
    H. Assess patient pretreatment and preheparinization for possible internal bleeding
    I. Monitor patient throughout treatment; do not leave patient unattended

11. If blood loss occurs
    A. Stop bleeding at any site
        (1) apply pressure to bleeding site
        (2) immediately turn off blood pump, clamp both sides of separated blood line or catheter
    B. Return blood in the extracorporeal circuit to the patient when appropriate
    C. Notify physician or advanced practice nurse
    D. Administer oxygen if blood loss is significant
    E. Obtain hemoglobin and hematocrit
    F. If blood loss is significant, administer IV fluids, volume expander, or transfuse as ordered

Patient Teaching

Before teaching begins, consider health literacy and individualize the approach by considering patient's cultural and health beliefs, preferences, and wishes

Treatment and Equipment-related Complications

1. Educate patient regarding
   A. Hemodialysis
      (1) principles
      (2) hemodialysis equipment, setup, and monitoring as appropriate for his/her level of self-care
      (3) hemodialysis procedure
   B. Anticoagulation therapy
      (1) rationale
      (2) drug
      (3) purpose
      (4) prescribed dose
      (5) route
      (6) possible complications
      (7) report any surgical, dental, or other procedures
      (8) onset of menses
      (9) other conditions that will require reevaluation of anticoagulation therapy
   C. Dialyzer reprocessing procedures and need for checking for the absence of sterilant in the dialyzer
   D. Signs and symptoms of treatment and equipment-related complications that should be promptly reported to staff
   E. Patient role in ensuring safe delivery and effectiveness of treatment
      (1) effects of position change, movement, and eating during treatment
      (2) measures that can be taken by the patient to prevent treatment and equipment-related complications
         a. ensure that proper dialyzer is being used
         b. check name on reprocessed dialyzer if in reuse program
         c. report of subjective interdialytic and intradialytic complaints
         d. ensure access site and extracorporeal connections remain uncovered during the treatment

> Report any surgical, dental, or other procedures; onset of menses; or other conditions that will require reevaluation of anticoagulation therapy

Advanced Practice Nursing Care
(In addition to items outlined above)

Assessment
1. Interpret results of diagnostic studies (e.g., laboratory tests, electrocardiogram [EKG], BVM profile, type, slope, and degree of plasma refill)
2. Evaluate patient response to treatment, including any treatment and equipment-related complications
3. Collaborate with interdisciplinary team in analysis of root causes of treatment and equipment-related complications
4. Review patient's medications prior to selecting or changing dialyzer

Intervention
1. Order laboratory tests and diagnostic studies as appropriate
2. Initiate interventions for treatment and equipment-related complications as necessary
3. Modify hemodialysis prescription based upon patient response to treatment and occurrence of complications
4. Order appropriate follow-up of complications

References
Association for the Advancement of Medical Instrumentation – www.aami.org/standards
Counts, C. (Ed.). (2008). *Core curriculum for nephrology nursing* (5th ed.). Pitman, NJ: American Nephrology Nurses' Association.

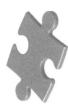

Patient Management

Patient Outcomes

The patient will receive a safe and appropriate dialysis treatment.

The patient will demonstrate knowledge of the hemodialysis procedure and treatment prescription.

The patient will be free of intradialytic morbidities.

The patient will meet or exceed targets for clinical performance measures.

Nursing Care

Assessment

1. Assess the patient predialysis, intradialysis, and postdialysis
   A. Weight
      (1) weight gain or loss
      (2) estimated dry weight compared to predialysis weight and last postdialysis weight
   B. Degree of ultrafiltration and ultrafiltration rate related to weight, age, and comorbidities that may affect safe fluid removal
   C. Temperature and changes between predialysis and postdialysis
   D. Blood pressure (sitting and standing) predialysis, intradialysis, and postdialysis
   E. Dose, type, timing, and continued need for BP medications (if patient held or took them pretreatment)
   F. Heart rate and sounds: apical and peripheral pulses (quality, rate, rhythm)
   G. Respiratory rate and quality, breath sounds, oxygen needs
   H. Neck vein distention, jugular venous pressure
   I. Capillary refill
   J. Condition and patency of vascular access (see Vascular Access section)
   K. Intake: oral, parenteral, intradialytic fluid intake
   L. Output including all fluid losses related to residual urine output, draining wounds, nasogastric tube, fever, diarrhea, ileostomy, diaphoresis, hyperventilation, and ultrafiltration
   M. Extravasation of fluids related to bowel dysfunction, ascites, and lymphocele
   N. Amount of urine output per 24 hours
   O. Response to and continued need for diuretics
   P. Dietary and fluid allowance prescription, appetite changes, and adherence to prescription
   Q. Sodium intake: source and amount
   R. Medication regimen and types/adherence
   S. Dialysate type, composition, temperature
   T. Continuous electrocardiogram (EKG) and pulse oximetry monitoring in children <20 kg; adults as indicated
   U. Blood volume monitoring (BVM) in children <35 kg; adults as indicated to establish, maintain, and reassess dry weight and assist in prevention and root cause of intradialytic symptoms
      (1) BVM profile type
      (2) slope
      (3) degree of plasma refill at end of treatment
      (4) bioimpedance spectroscopy

Patient Management

V. Assess the patient for ecchymoses, hematomas, or other signs of bleeding

W. Elicit history of injuries, bleeding, unusual bruising, menses, and surgical procedures

2. Assess the patient's general condition before, during, and after treatment
   A. Edema
      (1) facial
      (2) periorbital
      (3) hands
      (4) vascular access
      (5) peripheral: feet and ankles
      (6) sacral
      (7) abdominal: changes in abdominal girth measurement
   B. Skin and mucous membranes
      (1) turgor
      (2) color
         a. dusky
         b. pale
         c. flushing
         d. any change from normal color
   C. Mental status
      (1) orientation
      (2) confusion
      (3) restlessness
      (4) mood
      (5) any changes
   D. Ability to ambulate; gait changes
   E. General sense of well-being
   F. Level of functioning
   G. Any changes from baseline
   H. Reported recovery time posttreatment

Review available laboratory test results prior to initiation of treatment

3. Solicit symptoms and complaints from patient and evaluate prior to initiation of treatment, during treatment, and prior to discharge from facility
   A. Headache, dizziness, or blurred vision
   B. Nausea, vomiting
   C. Diarrhea, constipation, or tarry stool
   D. Fever, chills
   E. Shortness of breath, dyspnea
   F. Chest pain or palpitations
   G. Pain
   H. Bleeding
   I. Urgency or frequency of urination
   J. Insomnia
   K. Weakness, fatigue, or change in level of activity
   L. Change in appetite
   M. Degree of thirst
   N. Recovery time posttreatment

4. Review available laboratory test results prior to initiation of treatment
   A. Blood urea nitrogen (BUN) and serum creatinine, Kt/V, or URR
   B. Electrolytes: calcium, magnesium, potassium
   C. Hemoglobin, hematocrit, iron indices
   D. Phosphorus PTH level

Patient Management

E. Albumin

F. Atrial: brain nutriuretic peptides if available

G. Acid-base balance/Serum CO_2 level

H. Serum sodium and sodium set point

I. Serum glucose and glycosylated hemoglobin

J. Carnitine level

K. Angiotension level

L. Residual kidney function

5. Assess patient for symptoms and root cause of hypervolemia vs. hypovolemia

A. Interdialytic

   (1) hypertension

   (2) respiratory difficulties: shortness of breath, dyspnea on exertion, orthopnea

   (3) edema

   (4) feeling of abdominal fullness

   (5) GI symptoms: nausea, vomiting, diarrhea, changes in appetite

   (6) thirst level, changes

   (7) orthostatic hypotension, light-headedness, dizziness

   (8) weakness, fatigue

   (9) muscle cramping

   (10) decreases in urinary output

   (11) reported recovery time post reatment

B. Intradialytic

   (1) hypertension

   (2) hypotension

   (3) tachycardia, arrhythmia

   (4) chest pain

   (5) nausea, vomiting

   (6) dizziness, changes in sensorium, seizures

   (7) vision changes

   (8) muscle cramping

   (9) hypoxemia

Assess patient's psychosocial adjustment to hemodialysis

6. In addition to the above, assess the patient during the treatment for any of the following

A. Blood pressure and pulse outside of established parameters

B. Respiratory rate and quality outside of established parameters

C. Temperature

   (1) outside of established parameters

   (2) increase from pretemperature

D. Any new complaint reported by patient

E. Change in mental status (e.g., agitation, confusion)

F. Hemodialysis access

   (1) needles and connections secured

   (2) needles and connections visible at all times

   (3) difficulty with cannulation

   (4) infiltration or hematoma

   (5) unable to achieve or maintain prescribed blood flow rate

   (6) arterial or venous pressure outside of established parameters

   (7) bleeding

   (8) pain

7. Assess patient's response to the delivery of the hemodialysis prescription

Patient Management

8. Assess patient's psychosocial adjustment to hemodialysis
9. Assess patient's understanding of the hemodialysis procedure
10. Assess patient's immunization requirements

Intervention

1. Notify the physician or advanced practice nurse of any assessment finding or patient's response to the treatment that might require modification of the hemodialysis prescription
2. Adjust and administer prescribed hemodialysis treatment based on previous postassessment, predialysis assessment findings, interdialytic complaints, and postdialysis assessment
3. Maintain a dialysis log summarizing relevant information that provides a longitudinal dynamic view of extracellular volume and blood pressure changes such as body weight, blood pressure, and intradialysis symptoms; if available, BVM profile, type, slope, degree of plasma refill, and bioimpedance spectroscopy should be included
4. Review dialysis prescription and patient response with interdisciplinary team to determine appropriate individualized UF goal, related patient medical history, dialysis time, frequency, dialysate conductivity, temperature, and pH to promote optimal fluid management and minimize complications
5. Administer oxygen to prevent symptoms of and treat hypoxemia
6. Blood volume monitoring in children <35kg
7. Reevaluate medical justification for and avoid or eliminate intradialytic administration of sodium (oral, parenteral, dialysate) whenever possible
8. Reevaluate residual urine output at least quarterly; review for need to adjust or discontinue diuretics
9. Administer and monitor fluids according to prescribed treatment plan
10. Encourage adherence to prescribed sodium, fluid, and dietary regimens
11. Encourage adherence to medication regimen
12. Administer medications as prescribed; review for potential changes and possible causes of intradialysis and interdialysis symptoms
13. Replace blood volume mL for mL in neonates (e.g., replace volume of blood drawn for laboratory testing)
14. Provide or encourage diversional activity as appropriate
15. Encourage adherence to treatment regimen and provide ongoing skill development and support
16. Identify resources to assist patient to achieve fluid management goals, psychosocial adjustment, and rehabilitation goals
17. Initiate consultations or referrals as appropriate

Identify resources to assist patient to achieve fluid management goals, psychosocial adjustment, and rehabilitation goals

Patient Teaching

Before teaching begins, consider health literacy and individualize the approach by considering patient's cultural and health beliefs, preferences, and wishes

1. Instruct patient regarding
   A. Kidney function
   B. Hemodialysis principles
   C. Hemodialysis procedure
   D. Current treatment prescription
   E. Signs and symptoms of complications
   F. Blood pressure and its relationship to fluid management
   G. Anticoagulation

Patient Management

H. Vascular access (see Vascular Access section)
I. Laboratory tests
   (1) frequency
   (2) purpose
   (3) target goals
J. Monitoring of hemodialysis adequacy
K. Medication regimen, especially as impacted by dialysis treatments
L. Diet and fluid prescription
   (1) sodium restriction and thirst management
   (2) dietary and intradialytic sources of sodium; reading of food labels
   (3) relationship of serum glucose level to thirst
   (4) daily fluid allowance in relationship to urinary output
   (5) qualification of "fluid" food sources
   (6) recommended weight gains in between treatments
   (7) recommended UFR related to age, weight, dialysis time, and comorbidities
M. Reporting of symptoms, illnesses, injuries, bleeding, or hospitalizations since last treatment
N. Reporting of any medication changes (prescription and over-the-counter) since last treatment
O. Emergency procedures while on hemodialysis and interdialytic
P. Home monitoring of weight and BP measurement
Q. Parameters to take or hold BP medications before and after dialysis
R. Teach or reinforce the benefits of following the prescription for treatment, medication, exercise, and nutrition therapy
S. Importance of immunizations

Adjust the hemodialysis prescription based on patient's response to treatment

Advanced Practice Nursing Care

(In addition to items outlined above)

Assessment

1. Interpret results of diagnostic studies (e.g., laboratory tests, EKG, x-rays, echocardiogram, residual kidney function, BVM profile, type, slope, and degree of plasma refill, and bioimpedance spectroscopy)
2. Monitor patient's adherence to treatment plan
3. Monitor patient's response to the dialysis prescription
4. Monitor patient's response to medications and immunizations
5. Monitor patient's response to diet, sodium, and fluid prescriptions
6. Assess patient's dialysis access for complications
7. Review hospitalization admitting diagnosis for accuracy
8. Analyze dialysis log summarizing longitudinal dynamic view of extracellular volume and blood pressure changes
9. Coordinate root cause analysis of intradialytic morbidities

Intervention

1. Adjust the hemodialysis prescription based on patient's response to treatment. Modify
  A. Time
  B. Frequency
  C. Ultrafiltration goal and rate for patient age, size, dialysis time, and comorbidities
  D. Dialysate conductivity and pH
  E. Temperature

Patient Management

2. Order diagnostic studies as appropriate: laboratory tests, EKG, chest x-ray, echocardiogram, sleep studies, residual kidney function, and BVM type, slope, and plasma refill checks
3. Adjust diet and fluid prescription based on patient response
4. Adjust medication regimen based on patient response
    A. Adjust or remove antihypertensive agents as indicated
    B. Diuretic adjustments as indicated if urinary output is >100mL/qd
    C. Educate patient on immunization protocols
    D. Adjust erythropoiesis-stimulating agents, iron and bone disease medications as appropriate based on laboratoy results
5. Initiate treatment of dialysis access complications
6. Adjust sodium, fluid, and dietary prescriptions based on assessment of patient's response to treatment
7. Reevaluate target dry weight as needed
8. Order longer or extra treatment if medically justified to attain dry weight

References

Centers for Medicare and Medicaid Services. (2008). Conditions for coverage for end stage renal disease facilities: Final rule, Federal Register. Retrieved from http://www.cms.gov/cfcsandcops/downloads/esrdfinalrule0415.pdf

Counts, C. (Ed.). (2008). *Core curriculum for nephrology nursing* (5th ed). Pitman, NJ: American Nephrology Nurses' Association.

National Kidney Foundation. (2006b). NKF-KDOQI clinical practice guidelines for blood pressure management and use of antihypertensive agents in chronic kidney disease. *American Journal of Kidney Diseases, 48*(1)(Suppl. 1), S1-183.

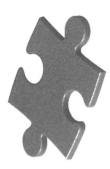

Peritoneal Dialysis

Peritoneal dialysis (PD) is a treatment that uses the body's natural membrane for fluid and solute exchange. It is a gentle and well-tolerated method for a wide range of people with ESRD, from the very young to the very old. It can be used in either an acute setting as an intervention for acute kidney injury (AKI) or in a home setting for individuals with ESRD.

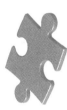

Catheter Implantation

Patient Outcomes

The PD catheter will function effectively and provide reasonable fill and drain flow rates.

The PD catheter will be free of complications and have a long-use life.

The patient will demonstrate knowledge regarding the PD catheter and its care.

Nursing Care

Assessment

1. Preoperative assessment of potential catheter insertion sites and exit sites
2. Integrity, patency, and function of the new PD catheter
3. Surgical incision and catheter exit site for healing
4. Catheter exit site for signs of early infection
5. Postoperative pain or discomfort
6. Postoperative complications
7. Effect of catheter on body image
8. Patient or partner's ability to perform dressing change procedures if indicated

Intervention

1. Participate in the decision regarding the preferred type and size of catheter
2. Participate in the decision regarding the catheter insertion site and placement of the exit site
3. Mark the exit site with indelible marker, as requested

Catheter Implantation

4. Obtain nasal or other cultures for determination of *S. aureus* carrier status
5. Administer prophylactic antibiotics as ordered
6. Irrigate the catheter intraoperatively as requested
7. Postoperatively, check that catheter is capped or connected securely to the sterile irrigation system
8. Irrigate catheter postoperatively or perform PD to maintain patency
9. Add anticoagulant to catheter "locking" solutions or dialysis solution
10. Perform postoperative dressing changes and exit site care

Patient Teaching

Before teaching begins, consider health literacy and individualize the approach by considering patient's cultural and health beliefs, preferences, and wishes

1. Teach the patient about the PD catheter
   A. Type of catheter
   B. Anticipated location of the catheter
   C. The surgical procedure
   D. Typical degree of pain or discomfort and interventions
   E. Normal progression of healing
   F. Activity restrictions to avoid high intraabdominal pressure during healing
   G. Bowel hygiene to avoid constipation
2. Teach patient to care for the new catheter
   A. Avoiding catheter movement and tension on the catheter
   B. Avoiding activities that raise intraabdominal pressure
   C. Postoperative dressing changes, exit site care, and catheter immobilization if applicable
   D. Restrictions related to showering and bathing
   E. Importance of continuing prophylactic antibiotic therapy if applicable
3. Signs and symptoms of infection and malfunction and importance of prompt reporting
4. Discuss effect of PD catheter on body image

References

Gokal, R., Alexander, S., Ash, S., Chen, T.W., Danielson, A., Holmes, C., Joffe, P., Moncrief, J., Nichols, K., Piraino, B., Prowant, B., Slingeneyer, A., Stegmayr, B., Twardowski, Z., & Vas, S. (1998). Peritoneal catheters and exit-site practices toward optimum peritoneal access: 1998 update. *Peritoneal Dialysis International, 18*(1), 11-33.

Twardowski, Z.J., & Prowant, B.F. (1996). Appearance and classification of healing peritoneal catheter exit sites. *Peritoneal Dialysis International, 16*(Suppl. 3), S71-S93.

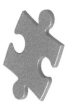

Acute Peritoneal Dialysis

Patient Outcomes

The patient will receive safe and effective peritoneal dialysis.

Nursing Care

Assessment

1. Primary kidney disease and comorbid conditions

Acute Peritoneal Dialysis

    2. Response to prior PD treatments
    3. Assess patient for
        A. Vital signs (pretherapy and posttherapy and at defined intervals throughout therapy)
            (1) supine and upright blood pressure
            (2) apical pulse rate and rhythm
            (3) rate and depth of respirations
        B. Fluid status
            (1) weight
            (2) intake and output, including parenteral infusions if appropriate
            (3) presence of edema
            (4) jugular venous distention
            (5) other hemodynamic parameters as applicable
    4. Level of consciousness
    5. Discomfort or pain
    6. Catheter type and implantation date
    7. Catheter dressing intact and dry
    8. Medication history
    9. Response to therapy
  10. Catheter malfunction
  11. Procedure-related complications
        A. Bleeding
        B. Pain or discomfort
            (1) abdominal discomfort
            (2) back pain
            (3) shoulder pain
            (4) rectal or suprapubic pressure or pain
        C. Dialysate leak
        D. Hernia
        E. Hemorrhoids
        F. Gastroesophageal reflux
        G. Acute hydrothorax
  12. Signs and symptoms of dialysis disequilibrium
        A. Headache
        B. Nausea and vomiting
        C. Hypertension
        D. Decreased sensorium
        E. Convulsions
        F. Coma
  13. Patient's and family's knowledge and understanding of the PD procedure
  14. Laboratory test results
        A. Urea and creatinine
        B. Albumin
        C. Potassium
        D. Bicarbonate
        E. Glucose
        F. Hemoglobin and hematocrit
        G. White blood count
        H. Platelets

Assess patient's and family's knowledge and understanding of the PD procedure

Acute Peritoneal Dialysis

15. Assess PD system
    A. Equipment
       (1) functioning appropriately
       (2) disinfected per protocol
       (3) disposable lines and tubings appropriate for machine
    B. Settings for exchange volume, drain, and fill times match prescription
    C. Dialysis solution and additives match prescription
    D. Alarms are set and functioning properly
    E. Connections are secure
    F. Closed system is intact without leaks
16. Assess dialysate
    A. Flow rate
    B. Drain volumes
    C. Solution color and clarity
17. Observe for complications of PD therapy

Intervention

1. Obtain blood, dialysate, and other samples for monitoring (pretreatment, during treatment, and after treatment)
2. Prepare equipment and dialysis solutions and initiate therapy
3. Secure connections between the catheter or transfer set and dialysis tubing
4. Use aseptic technique to add medications to the PD solution
5. Use aseptic technique for connection to and disconnection from the PD system
6. Monitor dialysis solution temperature
7. For patient with newly implanted catheter
    A. Dialyze in supine position
    B. Begin with low volumes and gradually increase exchange volume
    C. Add heparin to dialysis solutions as ordered
    D. Avoid activities that increase intraabdominal pressure
    E. Avoid constipation
8. Maintain a record of intake and output, including dialysis losses
9. Monitor potassium levels and add potassium to the dialysis solution as indicated
10. Assist patient with position changes if necessary to facilitate drainage
11. Provide comfort measures
12. Teach nurses appropriate monitoring and problem-solving techniques related to the PD therapy
13. Give postdialysis report to unit nurse responsible for the patient's care

Use aseptic technique for connection to and disconnection from the PD system

Patient Teaching

Before teaching begins, consider health literacy and individualize the approach by considering patient's cultural and health beliefs, preferences, and wishes

1. PD system
    A. Cycler or manual system
    B. Treatment-related procedures
    C. Monitoring
2. Explain the peritoneal dialysis procedure
3. Exchange cycle
    A. How PD works to remove wastes and fluid
    B. Anticipated length of treatment
4. Risks and complications associated with PD therapy

5. Signs and symptoms of treatment-related complications that should be reported promptly to the nurse
6. After dialysis, review dietary and fluid prescription orders

Reference

Korbet, S. M., & Kronfol, N.O. (2001). Acute peritoneal dialysis prescription. In J.T. Daugirdas, P.G. Blake, & T.S. Ing. (Eds.), *Handbook of dialysis* (3rd ed., pp. 333-342). Philadelphia: Lippincott Williams & Wilkins.

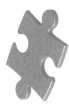

Dialysis Prescription and Adequacy

Patient Outcomes

The dialysis modality and prescription will be appropriate for the patient's size and peritoneal transport characteristics.

The patient will meet target goals for PD adequacy.

Nursing Care

Assessment

1. Peritoneal transport characteristics
2. Monitor level of residual renal function
3. Patient's understanding of the dialysis prescription
4. Patient's adherence to the dialysis prescription
5. Patient's understanding of adequacy-related concepts
   A. Importance of dialysis adequacy
   B. Relationship of dialysis prescription to dialysis adequacy
   C. Contribution of residual renal function to dialysis adequacy
   D. Outcomes associated with inadequate dialysis
   E. Dialysis adequacy collection procedures
   F. Any changes in dialysis prescription
6. Evaluation of accuracy of adequacy test results
   A. Typical dialysis regimen on collection day
   B. Completeness of dialysate and urine collections
   C. Accuracy of volume measurement and sampling
   D. Accurate weight and height used in calculations
   E. Correct formulas used and calculations accurate
7. Evaluation of dialysis adequacy
   A. Clinical assessment of dialysis adequacy
      (1) patient should look good and feel well
      (2) absence of anorexia and dysgeusia
      (3) absence of nausea and vomiting
      (4) absence of or improvement in weakness
      (5) absence of or improvement in fatigue
      (6) absence of or improvement in insomnia, sleep disorders
      (7) subjective global assessment of nutritional status

**Dialysis
Prescription**

B. Satisfactory subjective health-related quality of life (KDQOL or SF 36)

C. Determine if Kt/V(urea) and weekly creatinine clearance meet target values

D. Monitor residual renal function and its contribution to dialysis adequacy

E. Review normalized protein catabolic rate (nPCR) if available

8. Review peritoneal transport characteristic results to guide changes in modality or prescription

9. If the delivered dialysis dose is below the target level, evaluate cause

A. Inadequate prescription

B. Lack of adherence to prescription

C. Change in peritoneal transport

D. Loss of residual renal function

Intervention

1. Perform tests to determine peritoneal transport characteristics

2. Take measures to preserve residual renal function (see Universal Guidelines, Residual Kidney Function)

3. Obtain dialysate and urine collection or samples and related information from patient; process for laboratory

4. Report adequacy results to the physician or advanced practice nurse

5. Discuss dialysis prescription changes with the physician or advanced practice nurse if indicated

6. Enhance CAPD dialysis prescription by increasing exchange volume and/or number of exchanges

7. Enhance automated PD (or CCPD) prescription by adding a day dwell, increasing dwell volumes, adding cycler time, or increasing the number of cycles

8. Repeat adequacy testing if indicated

9. Relay any prescription changes to the patient

10. Refer to dietitian if nPCR is low or low protein intake is a problem

Patient Teaching

Before teaching begins, consider health literacy and individualize the approach by considering patient's cultural and health beliefs, preferences, and wishes

1. Provide both verbal and written instructions and supplies required for 24-hour collections of dialysate and urine

2. Explain the relationship of the dialysis prescription to dialysis adequacy

3. Emphasize the contribution of residual renal function and urine volume to dialysis adequacy

4. Review adequacy test results with the patient

5. Review and explain any changes in dialysis prescription

6. Explain rationale for components of dialysis prescription

Emphasize the contribution of residual renal function and urine volume to dialysis adequacy

References

Blake, P.G., & Diaz-Buxo, J. (2001). Adequacy of peritoneal dialysis and chronic peritoneal dialysis prescription. In J.T. Daugirdas, P.G. Blake, & T.S. Ing. (Eds.), *Handbook of dialysis* (3rd ed., pp. 343-360). Philadelphia: Lippincott Williams & Wilkins.

National Kidney Foundation. (2001). K/DOQI clinical practice guidelines for peritoneal dialysis adequacy. *American Journal of Kidney Diseases, 37*(1)(Suppl. 1), S65-S136.

Oreopoulos, D.G., & Rao, P. (2001). Assessing peritoneal ultrafiltration, solute transport, and volume status. In J.T. Daugirdas, P.G. Blake, & T.S. Ing. (Eds.), *Handbook of dialysis* (3rd ed., pp. 361-372). Philadelphia: Lippincott Williams & Wilkins.

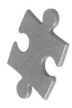

Prevention and Treatment of Complications

Common complications include bleeding, hyperglycemia, catheter malfunction, and infectious complications.

Patient Outcomes

The patient will be free from complications related to peritoneal dialysis.

The home dialysis patient will identify and report PD-related problems appropriately.

The patient will participate in the management of PD-related problems.

BLEEDING

Patient Outcome

The patient will not experience complications related to intraperitoneal bleeding.

Nursing Care

Assessment

1. Monitor for the presence of blood in the dialysate
2. Assess for the etiology of bleeding
   A. Medical or surgical procedures
   B. Trauma
   C. Ovulation or menstruation
   D. Infection
3. Evaluate the extent of bleeding
   A. Color of dialysate
   B. Comparison of dialysate color over a series of exchanges
   C. Hematocrit of dialysate in severe bleeding
   D. Systemic signs of bleeding and hypovolemia
4. Determine if the patient has received systemic anticoagulation therapy

Intervention

1. Inform the nephrologist or advanced practice nurse if there is more than minimal bleeding (frank red dialysate)
2. Add heparin to the dialysis solution to prevent clotting in the catheter, as ordered or per protocol
3. Rapid exchanges with room temperature dialysis solution

Prevention and Treatment – Bleeding

Patient Teaching

Before teaching begins, consider health literacy and individualize the approach by considering patient's cultural and health beliefs, preferences, and wishes

1. For the acute dialysis patient
   A. Etiology of bleeding if known
   B. Reason for monitoring
   C. Anticipated course
   D. Interventions
2. For the home patient
   A. Routine monitoring for bleeding
   B. Evaluating the extent of bleeding
   C. When to report bleeding
   D. Possible causes of intraperitoneal bleeding
   E. Adding heparin to the dialysis solution
      (1) drug, concentration, dose, and frequency
      (2) technique for adding intraperitoneal medications

HYPERGLYCEMIA

Patient Outcome

The patient will maintain glycemic control during the peritoneal dialysis treatment.

Nursing Care

Assessment

For acute patients
1. Determine if there is a prior history of diabetes mellitus, hyperglycemia, or glucose intolerance
2. Review type and dose of antidiabetic medications
3. Evaluate blood glucose results and compare to values prior to the initiation of PD therapy
4. Observe for signs and symptoms of hyperglycemia and hypoglycemia

For home patients
1. Review laboratory results, specifically glucose levels and glycosylated hemoglobin
2. Home records
   A. Use of hypertonic dialysis solutions
   B. Frequency of blood glucose testing
   C. Glucose levels and insulin doses
   D. Other antidiabetic agents
3. Determine the effect of dialysis solution composition on serum glucose
4. Query regarding hyperglycemic and hypoglycemic episodes
5. Assess patient's or caregiver's ability to
   A. Monitor glucose
   B. Make decisions regarding glucose management
   C. Administer insulin properly
6. Check that home glucose monitoring devices have been calibrated

Prevention and Treatment – Hyperglycemia

Intervention

1. Monitor blood glucose during acute dialysis as ordered or per protocol
2. Notify nephrologist or advanced practice nurse of abnormal blood glucose results in acute dialysis patients
3. Administer antidiabetic agents as ordered, including intraperitoneal insulin
4. Confer with physician or advanced practice nurse regarding changes in dialysis regimen
5. Confer with physician, advanced practice nurse, or diabetologist for changes in antidiabetic agents or insulin regimen
6. Initiate dietary consult for acute patients if indicated
7. Request dietary teaching for chronic patients if indicated

Patient Teaching

Before teaching begins, consider health literacy and individualize the approach by considering patient's cultural and health beliefs, preferences, and wishes

1. Effect of peritoneal dialysis on blood glucose in patients with diabetes and those with glucose intolerance
2. Effect of dialysis solution dextrose concentration on blood glucose in patients with diabetes and those with glucose intolerance
3. Parameters for use of hypertonic solutions
4. Purpose of glucose monitoring
5. Home glucose monitoring procedure and documentation
6. Signs and symptoms of hyperglycemia and hypoglycemia
7. Goals for glucose control
8. Glucose and glycosylated hemoglobin results
9. Changes in type or dose of antidiabetic agents
10. Procedure to add insulin to dialysis solutions, if intraperitoneal insulin is ordered

CATHETER MALFUNCTION

Patient Outcome

The PD catheter will function effectively and provide reasonable fill and drain flow rates.

The PD catheter will have a long use life.

Nursing Care

Assessment

1. Observe catheter fill and drain flow rates
2. Document inability to infuse or drain
3. Check catheter and tubings for external clamps, kinks, or pressure
4. Inspect tubings for air bubbles that may cause an "air lock"
5. For gravity-driven systems
   A. Check height of dialysis solution bags above abdomen
   B. Check distance from lowest point of peritoneal cavity to drain bag
6. Determine if drain flow problems are related to patient position
7. Observe for fibrin or blood clots in dialysate
8. Determine if patient is constipated

Prevention and Treatment – Catheter Malfunction

9. Document catheter position by x-ray
10. Review results of abdominal x-rays (flat plate and lateral views) for internal kink in catheter

Intervention

1. Adjust height of dialysis solution bags to enhance drain and fill rates
2. Change patient's position to enhance dialysate drain rates or to obtain complete drain
3. Add heparin to dialysis or irrigation solutions
4. Infuse solution under pressure or irrigate catheter manually with a large syringe in an attempt to
   A. Dislodge blood or fibrin clots
   B. Flush air bubbles out of the tubing and catheter
5. Perform or assist with procedure to manually remove clots from catheter
6. For malpositioned catheter
   A. Encourage or assist with ambulation and activity
   B. Have patient assume a knee-chest position in an attempt to reposition catheter
   C. Induce peristalsis
   D. Assist with medical procedure to manually reposition catheter
7. Administer thrombolytics if ordered
8. Induce peristalsis or a bowel movement if patient is constipated
9. Initiate or request consultations or referrals as indicated
10. Consult with physician or advanced practice nurse regarding necessity of surgical intervention

Patient Teaching

Before teaching begins, consider health literacy and individualize the approach by considering patient's cultural and health beliefs, preferences, and wishes

1. Instruct the home patient
   A. To check for clamps, kinks, or pressure on the catheter or tubings
   B. To observe for blood or fibrin clots
   C. How to add heparin to the dialysis solution when clots are observed
   D. To raise or lower bags to enhance flow by gravity
   E. To change position to enhance flows if indicated
   F. Review strategies to avoid or treat constipation
2. For acute catheter problems, explain
   A. The known or suspected etiology of the problem
   B. The nature of diagnostic tests and intervention procedures

INFECTIOUS COMPLICATIONS

Peritonitis remains a leading complication of peritoneal dialysis. Many of the general principles can be applied to pediatric patients. The recommendations outlined here reflect care of the adult peritoneal patient. Terminology for peritonitis is located in Table 4.2.

Patient Outcomes

The patient will not have catheter-related infection or peritonitis.

The patient will recognize signs and symptoms of infectious complications and will report infection promptly.

Nursing Care

Assessment

1. For peritonitis
   A. Dialysate
      (1) turbidity
      (2) presence of fibrin
      (3) color
      (4) presence of fecal material
   B. Query patient regarding subjective symptoms and onset of episode
   C. Presence of concurrent exit site and tunnel infection
   D. History of known contamination or break in technique
   E. Recent invasive procedures
   F. Laboratory results
      (1) culture and sensitivity
      (2) cell count with differential

Table 4.2	
Terminology for Peritonitis 2010 ISPD Guidelines/Recommendations	
Recurrent	An episode that occurs within 4 weeks of completion of therapy of a prior episode but with a different organism
Relapsing	An episode that occurs within 4 weeks of completion of therapy of a prior episode with the same organism or one sterile episode
Repeat	An episode that occurs within 4 weeks of completion of therapy of a prior episode with the organism
Refractory	Failure of the effluent to clear 5 days of appropriate antibiotics
Catheter-related peritonitis	Peritonitis in conjunction with an exit-site or tunnel infection with the same organism or one site sterile

Prevention and Treatment – Infectious Complications

    G. Abdominal pain
        (1) Abdominal pain with clear fluid: assess for constipation renal of biliary colic, peptic ulcer disease, pancreatitis
  2. For exit site infection: infection of an exit site may be indicated by purulent drainage; erythema may or may not indicate an infection. A tunnel infection may present as erythema, edema, or tenderness over the subcutaneous pathway
    A. Inspection of external exit site and visible tunnel for signs of infection
        (1) erythema
        (2) induration
        (3) large crust or scab
        (4) drainage
            a. purulent
            b. serosanguinous
        (5) exuberant granulation tissue
    B. Query patient for subjective symptoms of infection
    C. *S. aureus* carrier status
    D. History of exit site trauma
    E. Culture and sensitivity
  3. Drug allergies
  4. Procedure technique if etiology of peritonitis is unknown
  5. Routine exit site care regimen
  6. Monitor response to treatment

Assess patient's understanding of infectious complications

Intervention

1. Use aseptic technique for all dialysis procedures
2. Follow unit protocols for postimplantation and chronic exit site care
3. Obtain order for prophylactic antibiotic therapy prior to invasive procedures (e.g., dental surgery, colonoscopy with biopsy)
4. Obtain dialysate samples for laboratory testing using aseptic technique
5. Obtain culture of exit site exudate if present; a swab of the exit site if there is no exudate
6. Administer antibiotics, pain medication, and heparin, as ordered
    A. Exit site infections are caused by a variety of organisms; *S. aureus* and *P. aeruginosa* are responsible for the majority of infections
7. Review laboratory reports and notify physician or advanced practice nurse of results
8. Schedule for follow-up evaluations
9. Schedule for retraining if appropriate
10. Notify physician or advanced practice nurse if signs and symptoms of infection persist
11. Regularly monitor infection rates
12. Assess patient's understanding of infectious complications

Patient Teaching

Before teaching begins, consider health literacy and individualize the approach by considering patient's cultural and health beliefs, preferences, and wishes

Prior to infection
1. Concepts of sterility, aseptic technique, and contamination
2. Safe PD connection, disconnection, and exchange procedures
3. Exit site care and use of prophylactic antibiotics (e.g., mupirocin calcium, gentamicin)
4. Exit site assessment and reporting of problems
5. Precautions related to swimming or submersion of the exit site
6. Importance of avoiding tension on the catheter and trauma to the exit site

Prevention and Treatment – Infectious Complications

7. Importance of aseptic technique in PD procedures and of following procedures exactly as taught
8. Contamination of the PD system
    A. Recognizing contamination
    B. Procedure for a break in the PD system
    C. Procedure for known contamination
    D. Importance of reporting suspected or known contamination
    E. Prophylactic antibiotic therapy if ordered
9. Signs and symptoms of PD-related infections
    A. Exit site infection
    B. Tunnel or cuff infection
    C. Peritonitis
10. Importance of reporting signs and symptoms of infection immediately
    A. Save drained cloudy dialysate and bring to the clinic

At diagnosis of infection
1. Medication regimen
    A. Route, dose, and frequency of drugs prescribed for the infection
    B. Signs and symptoms of an allergic reaction
    C. Technique for adding drugs to the dialysis solution if indicated
    D. Duration of therapy and importance of completing entire course of antibiotic therapy
2. Anticipated response to therapy
3. Signs and symptoms to monitor
4. Review principles of asepsis and procedure technique for patients with peritonitis of unknown etiology
5. Review exit site care procedure and assessment for patients with exit site or tunnel infections

References

Keane, W.F., Bailie, G.R., Boeschoten, E., Gokal, R., Golper, T.A., Holmes, C.J., Kawaguchi, Y., Piraino, B., Riella, M., & Vas, S. (2000). Adult peritoneal dialysis-related peritonitis treatment recommendations: 2000 Update. *Peritoneal Dialysis International, 20*(6), 828-829.

Kam-Tao, P., Szeto, C.C., Piraino, B., Bernardini, J., Figueiredo, A.E., Gupta, A., Johnson, D.W., Kuijper, E.J., Lye, W.C., Salzer, W, Schafer, F., & Struijk, D.G. (2010). Peritoneal dialysis-related infections recommendations: 2010 update. *Peritoneal Dialysis International, 30*, 393-423.

Twardowski, Z.J., & Prowant, B.F. (1996). Classification of normal and diseased exit sites. *Peritoneal Dialysis International, 16*(Suppl. 3), S32-S50.

Warady, B.A., Schaefer, F., Holloway, M., Alexander, S., Kandert, M., Piraino, B., Salusky, I., Tranaeus, A., Divino, J., Honda, M., Mujais, S., & Verrina, E. International Society for Peritoneal Dialysis (ISPD) Advisory Committee on Peritonitis Management in Pediatric Patients. (2000). Consensus guidelines for the treatment of peritonitis in pediatric patients receiving peritoneal dialysis. *Peritoneal Dialysis International, 20*(6), 610-624. Erratum in (2001). *Peritoneal Dialysis International, 21*(1), 6.

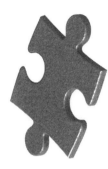

Self-Care and Home Dialysis

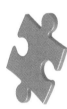

Evaluation and Education

Patient Outcomes

The patient will receive information regarding all modalities that are available and medically appropriate.

The patient will make an informed decision regarding treatment modality and setting.

The family of the pediatric patient will make an informed decision regarding treatment modality and setting.

Nursing Management

Assessment

1. Assess patient's knowledge of treatment options
    A. Hemodialysis
        (1) in-center
        (2) self-care, in-center
        (3) home dialysis
            a. nocturnal
            b. daily
    B. Peritoneal dialysis
        (1) continuous cycling peritoneal dialysis (CCPD)
        (2) continuous ambulatory peritoneal dialysis (CAPD)
    C. Transplantation
        (1) kidney, deceased donor
        (2) kidney, living donor
        (3) kidney–pancreas
2. Assess patient's degree of interest in and desire for a home dialysis modality or self-care in-center
3. In collaboration with the health care team and patient, evaluate
    A. Cognitive and psychomotor skills
    B. Spoken language
    C. Literacy level
    D. Ability to follow instructions
        (1) verbal
        (2) written
    E. Experience with and ability to follow treatment regimens
    F. If previously on dialysis, obtain dialysis history and evaluate patient's clinical stability during dialysis treatments

Evaluation and Education

G. Family relationships that may impact the overall success of home dialysis

H. Physical disabilities that may significantly limit the achievement of safe and effective treatments

4. Assess the home environment
   A. Cleanliness
   B. Local ordinances regarding waste disposal, building permits, etc.
   C. Electricity
   D. Water and plumbing
   E. Telephone access
   F. Space for supply storage and equipment

Intervention

1. Report findings to interdisciplinary team regarding patient interest in and desire for home or self-care dialysis
2. Report assessment of patient's abilities and limitations specific to the performance of home or self-care dialysis
3. Provide recommendations for home dialysis education and training
4. If the patient is not a candidate for home dialysis, provide recommendations for self-care education and skill building
5. Provide recommendations for any home modification required for home dialysis
6. Collaborate with health care team and patient to establish realistic goals for self-care or home dialysis
7. Collaborate with the health care team and patient to develop an educational plan that focuses on the necessary skills for self-care or home dialysis

Patient Teaching

Before teaching begins, consider health literacy and individualize the approach by considering patient's cultural and health beliefs, preferences, and wishes

1. Provide information regarding kidney replacement therapies; use techniques and materials appropriate for the patient's developmental stage, culture, and disabilities
   A. Hemodialysis
   B. Peritoneal dialysis
   C. Kidney transplantation
   D. Conservative management with palliative care
2. Dialysis modality education should include, but not be limited to
   A. Modality types and treatment settings
   B. Dialysis process and procedures
   C. Access types and placement
   D. Medications
   E. Advantages and disadvantages of each modality
   F. Expected outcomes
   G. Complications
   H. Lifestyle adaptation
   I. Rehabilitation potential
   J. Financial considerations
3. Transplant education should include, but not be limited to
   A. Definitions and types of transplants
   B. Evaluation process
   C. Surgical procedure
   D. Advantages and disadvantages
   E. Expected outcomes

Report findings to interdisciplinary team regarding patient interest in and desire for home or self-care dialysis

Evaluation and Education

F. Complications
G. Lifestyle adaptation
H. Rehabilitation potential
I. Financial considerations

4. Describe the purpose for the comprehensive evaluation
5. Discuss the timeline for the evaluation process
6. Explain the patient's and family's roles in the evaluation and decision processes
7. Describe the role of each health care team member in the evaluation and decision processes
8. Teach patient how to set goals and develop strategies to meet learning needs as appropriate

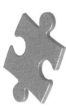

Dialysis Training

Patient Outcome

The patient will perform dialysis safely and effectively.

Nursing Care

Assessment

1. Identify patient and caregiver(s) who will be involved in home dialysis and training
2. Assess patient's current level of knowledge related to chronic kidney disease, diet, medications, current plan of care, and treatment goals
3. Determine patient's previous success with self-care
4. Assess patient's preferred method of learning (e.g., reading, watching, listening, performing)

Intervention

1. Involve patient and family in the development of an interdisciplinary teaching plan
2. Use culturally sensitive and ethnically appropriate educational materials
3. Use teaching techniques and materials that are appropriate for the patient's developmental stage and disabilities
4. Refer patient to additional resources that support or supplement the home dialysis or self-care education and training
5. Reinforce education and training using multiple approaches, including return demonstrations, verbal and written feedback
6. Promote age-appropriate self-care for pediatric patients
7. Encourage verbalization of anxieties, fears, and questions
8. Offer emotional support
9. Evaluate patient's learning by appropriate patient-specific testing
10. Ask patient to informally assess the instructor(s) on an ongoing basis
11. At completion of home dialysis training, obtain a formal evaluation of the training program using anonymous evaluation forms
12. Document in the medical record that the patient, the caregiver, or both, received and demonstrated adequate comprehension of the training

Dialysis Training

Patient Teaching

Training must be conducted by a registered nurse with at least 12 months of experience in providing nursing care and an additional 3 months of experience in the specific modality for which the nurse will provide self-care training

1. Discuss learning objectives, expected duration of training, and criteria for successful completion
2. Explain that additional teaching materials may be provided at later visits, but basic principles and skills will be stressed during initial training
3. Taking into consideration the patient's preferred method of learning, implement a teaching plan that includes, but is not limited to
    A. Review of kidney function
        (1) normal function
        (2) altered function in diseased kidneys
    B. Modality review
    C. Principles of dialysis
        (1) definitions
        (2) processes
        (3) access function
        (4) benefits
        (5) complications and risks
        (6) lifestyle adaptations
        (7) nutritional considerations
        (8) mobility and activity
        (9) financial considerations
    D. Infection control concepts
        (1) asepsis
        (2) handwashing
        (3) barrier protection
        (4) treatment environment
        (5) appropriate location for treatment
        (6) prevention of infections
        (7) prophylactic treatment of contamination of the PD system
        (8) prophylactic treatment for severe exit site trauma in PD patients
        (9) importance of following procedures for access care
        (10) situations that may increase the risk of infection
        (11) disposal of contaminated supplies and dialysate
        (12) signs and symptoms of infection
    E. Home treatment
        (1) treatment schedule
        (2) procedures
        (3) effective administration of medications
            a. adding intravenous (IV) or intraperitoneal (IP) medications
        (4) management of problems and emergencies including reporting to the health care team
        (5) maintenance of home treatment records including submission to and review by the health care team
        (6) ordering and inventory of supplies
        (7) water system for home hemodialysis
        (8) equipment maintenance and disinfection
        (9) waste disposal

Taking into consideration the patient's preferred method of learning, implement a teaching plan

Dialysis Training

F. Dialysis access
    (1) routine care, cleansing, and dressing changes
    (2) routine assessment
    (3) disinfection and aseptic procedures to initiate and discontinue dialysis
    (4) signs and symptoms of complications
        a. infection
        b. thrombosis
    (5) how to detect, report, and manage potential dialysis complications, including water treatment problems

G. Anemia
    (1) tests to evaluate anemia
    (2) procedures for specimen collection
    (3) effective administration of erythropoiesis-stimulating agent(s) (if prescribed) to achieve and maintain a target level hemoglobin or hematocrit as written in patient's plan of care

H. Dialysis adequacy
    (1) tests to evaluate adequacy
    (2) procedures for specimen collection specific to therapy type
    (3) expected results or target values
    (4) changes in prescription based on test results

I. Routine laboratory and radiology tests
    (1) purpose
    (2) frequency
    (3) procedure for obtaining samples
    (4) acceptable or target values

Use of complementary and alternative medicines and treatments

J. Nutrition
    (1) nutritional requirements and limitations
        a. calories
        b. protein
        c. sodium and fluid
        d. potassium
        e. vitamins
        f. calcium and phosphorus
        g. fat intake
        h. simple sugars
    (2) incorporating diet prescription into lifestyle
    (3) shopping, food preparation, and dining out

K. Medications
    (1) identification and name
    (2) purpose
    (3) dosage
    (4) route of administration
    (5) side effects and precautions
    (6) drug interactions
    (7) relationship to dietary intake
    (8) instructions for missed dose
    (9) use of over-the-counter medications
    (10) use of complementary and alternative medicines and treatments

L. Psychosocial issues
    (1) emotional responses
    (2) body image
    (3) sexual function

Dialysis Training

    (4) exercise and physical activity

    (5) rehabilitation

    (6) counseling services

    (7) financial resources

    (8) patient organizations

M. Patient rights and responsibilities

    (1) informed consent

    (2) advance directives

    (3) plan of care

    (4) medical record

        a. access for patient review

        b. confidentiality

    (5) grievance mechanism

N. Communication with health care team members

    (1) telephone numbers

        a. nursing staff during business hours

        b. emergency, after hours contact numbers

        c. physician, advanced practice nurse

    (2) introduction and roles of team members

        a. nurse

        b. social worker

        c. dietitian

        d. others in facility

    (3) schedule

        a. clinic hours

        b. scheduling nonroutine appointments

        c. after hours coverage

O. Resources

    (1) publications

    (2) kidney-related organizations and agencies

    (3) peer counseling by other kidney patients

    (4) audiovisual materials

    (5) Internet information sites

    (6) ESRD classes and lectures

P. Emergency procedures

    (1) power failure

    (2) disaster planning

        a. What to do

        b. Where to go, including instructions for occasions when the geographic area must be evacuated

        c. Whom to contact if an emergency occurs, contact information to include an alternate emergency phone number for the facility for instances when the dialysis facility is unable to receive phone calls due to an emergency

        d. How to disconnect themselves from the dialysis machine if an emergency occurs

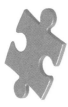

Ongoing Monitoring

Patient Outcomes

The patient will perform dialysis safely at home.

The patient will achieve and maintain a reasonable fluid balance.

Ongoing Monitoring

The patient will identify and report dialysis-related problems appropriately.

The patient will participate in the management of dialysis-related problems.

Nursing Care

Assessment

1. Vital signs, including supine and upright blood pressure
2. Degree of independence or assistance in performing dialysis procedures
3. Review home dialysis records, including computerized information for thoroughness and essential clinical parameters
4. Review glucose monitoring and insulin doses in patients with diabetes
5. Laboratory test results, including serum chemistry and hematology reports and special studies
6. Clinical response to dialysis therapy
   A. Dialysis adequacy measurements
   B. Fluid balance
      (1) ultrafiltration/fluid removal
      (2) achievement of dry weight
      (3) blood pressure control
   C. Intradialytic or interdialytic symptoms
7. Level of success in management of problems or emergencies
8. Vascular access patency and function
9. Assessment of catheter (HD and PD patients)
   A. Catheter integrity
   B. Catheter exit site and tunnel for signs and symptoms of infection
10. Outpatient medications, both prescribed and over-the-counter
11. Understanding of and adherence to prescribed diet
12. Reassess knowledge of
    A. Access site care
    B. Dialysis procedures
    C. Understanding of fluid balance
       (1) Weight and fluid balance goals
       (2) Role of fluid intake and dialysis in achieving fluid balance
       (3) Day-to-day assessment of fluid balance
    D. Knowledge of signs and symptoms of complications to report
13. Identify new learning needs with patient, caregiver, and/or family
14. Level of physical activity and exercise
15. Employment status or school attendance
16. Level of participation in family and community activities
17. Quality of life, subjective and measured
18. Satisfaction with therapy and burden of care for patient and family or caregiver
19. Assess for dialysis-related complications
20. Monitor the incidence of infectious complications
21. Development and periodic review of the patient's individualized comprehensive plan of care that specifies the services necessary to address the patient's needs and meets the measurable and expected outcomes

Intervention

1. Maintain regular contact with home patients
   A. By telephone

Monitor the incidence of infectious complications

B. Clinic visits every 4 to 6 weeks

   C. Home visits as needed; evaluate

      (1) treatment area

      (2) supply storage, organization, and inventory

      (3) dialysis procedure if indicated

      (4) patient's physical condition and activity level

      (5) family relationships and interactions

2. Provide guidance and support for home dialysis and self-care
3. Answer questions
4. Assist in problem solving
5. Assist in ordering supplies if necessary
6. Communicate and explain any changes in dialysis therapy
7. Schedule clinic visits, laboratory tests, and other diagnostic procedures
8. Provide a support system for problems or complications
9. Coordinate transition of treatment related information and care upon hospital admission and discharge
10. Report any changes in patient condition to appropriate health care team members
11. Assure appropriate follow-up

   A. By other members of the nephrology team

   B. For routine health care and screening

   C. By specialists, as indicated

Patient Teaching

Before teaching begins, consider health literacy and individualize the approach by considering patient's cultural and health beliefs, preferences, and wishes

1. Review and reinforce learning of critical components of home dialysis

   A. Access care

   B. Dialysis prescription

   C. Interpretation of dialysis adequacy test results

   D. Dialysis procedures and related skills

   E. Understanding of fluid balance

      (1) weight and fluid balance goals

      (2) role of fluid intake and dialysis solutions in achieving fluid balance

      (3) day-to-day assessment of fluid balance

      (4) knowledge of signs and symptoms of complications to report

   F. Medications

   G. Diet prescription

   H. Infection control

2. Treatment for infectious complications
3. Technique for adding intraperitoneal medications when IP drugs are ordered for PD patients
4. Changes in dialysis prescription
5. New devices, systems, procedures, or dialysis solutions
6. New medications
7. Evaluation strategies and interventions for dialysis and CKD complications
8. Topics specific to individual knowledge deficits
9. Continue to reinforce learning by

   A. Verbal feedback

   B. Return demonstration

   C. Testing as appropriate

Provide a support system for problems or complications

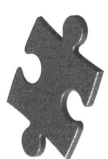

Apheresis and Therapeutic Plasma Exchange

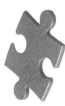

Pretreatment Patient Education

Patient Outcome

The patient will demonstrate knowledge of and ability to follow treatment regimen.

Nursing Care

Assessment

1. Assess patient's current level of knowledge
   A. Disease
   B. Diet
   C. Medications
   D. Current treatment plan
   E. Treatment procedure
   F. Preferred language and learning style: auditory, visual, written, tactile

Intervention

1. Involve support person or family in teaching process
2. Refer patient to other learning resources
3. Encourage verbalization of anxiety, fears, and questions
4. Provide emotional support
5. Provide culturally competent care

Pretreatment Patient Education

Patient Teaching

Before teaching begins, consider health literacy and individualize the approach by considering patient's cultural and health beliefs, preferences, and wishes

1. Implement a teaching plan that includes, but is not limited to
   A. Current clinical condition
   B. Rationale for treatment
   C. Overview of treatment procedure
   D. Vascular access type and care
   E. Potential benefits, risks, and complications
   F. Description of apheresis procedure
   G. For pediatric patients
      (1) "Does it hurt?"
      (2) "Can Mom or Dad stay?"
      (3) "How long does it take?"
   H. Dietary plan
   I. Medications
   J. Expected activity level during and after treatment
   K. Follow-up care
   L. Financial aspects
   M. Psychological aspects
   N. Advance directives

Reference

Counts, C. (Ed.). (2008). *Core curriculum for nephrology nurses* (5th ed., pp. 340-341). Pitman, NJ: American Nephrology Nurses' Association.

Patient Assessment

Patient Outcome

The patient will receive appropriate therapy and nursing care based on data from the patient assessment.

Nursing Care

Assessment

1. The treatment assessment is a total body systems review. The patient's past medical history and current status are assessed for each body system and disease-specific findings. Assessment should include, but not be limited to
   A. Temperature
   B. Cardiovascular status
      (1) blood pressure, sitting and standing when able
      (2) baseline electrocardiogram (EKG)
      (3) heart sounds
      (4) pulse rate, rhythm, and quality
      (5) peripheral pulses
      (6) age-appropriate parameters for growth and development in pediatric patients

Patient Assessment

C. Neurologic status
  (1) baseline mentation, orientation
  (2) mobility
  (3) sensation
  (4) cranial nerve function
  (5) bilateral strength
  (6) bilateral deep tendon or muscle reflexes
D. Respiratory system
  (1) bilateral breath sounds
  (2) respiratory rate and rhythm
  (3) oxygen saturation
  (4) pulmonary function test results if available
  (5) use of ancillary or abdominal muscles
  (6) presence of pulsus paradoxus or pulsus alternans
  (7) bronchial clearance
  (8) ability to speak and quality of speech
  (9) gag reflex
E. Gastrointestinal tract
  (1) nausea and vomiting
  (2) bowel sounds
  (3) elimination pattern
  (4) pain
F. Renal
  (1) function
    a. urine output
    b. BUN and creatinine serum levels
  (2) volume status
    a. intake and output
    b. presence or absence of edema
    c. weight
G. Integument
  (1) skin integrity, temperature, color, turgor
  (2) skin ulcerations, rashes, petechiae, ecchymoses, hematomas
H. Psychosocial
  (1) emotional status and coping mechanisms
  (2) sense of well-being
  (3) mental and physical functioning
  (4) patient and family understanding of illness and treatment
I. Current medication regimen
  (1) Angiotension-converting enzyme inhibitors (ACE-I) must be stopped 24–48 hours prior to treatment to prevent allergic and anaphylactic reactions
  (2) drugs that bind to plasma proteins may be removed during TPE
  (3) immunoglobulins may be removed during TPE
  (4) plasma cholinesterase is removed during TPE, creating anesthesia risk
  (5) vasopressors, pain meds, and continuous IV drips may need dose adjustments
  (6) TPE should follow rather than precede administration of infusions largely distributed in plasma (e.g., immunoglobulin, rituximab, monoclonal antibody, or antineoplastic medications)
J. Laboratory and test results for disease related serum assays are completed prior to first treatment
  (1) complete blood count with platelets

Plasma cholinesterase is removed during TPE, creating anesthesia risk

Patient Assessment

(2) fibrinogen level

(3) prothrombin time (PT), partial prothrombin time (PPT), international normalized ratio (INR)

(4) chemistry profile

(5) disease-specific laboratory analyses as appropriate

    a. daily CBC and lactate dehydrogenase (LDH) levels for patient with thrombotic thrombocytopenic purpura (TTP)

    b. immunoglobulin levels for Waldenstrom's macroglobulinemia or multiple myeloma

(6) hepatitis status

K. Vascular access

  (1) type

    a. catheter size and design to provide required flows for pediatric or adult patients with accommodation of size

    b. Permanent vascular access for maintenance (i.e., AV fistula/graft)

  (2) confirmation of appropriate placement

  (3) patency

  (4) condition of exit site or dressing

  (5) assess for complications of thrombosis, infection, aneurysms, venous hyptertension, seromas, bleeding

2. Compare data to previous findings

Intervention

Determine safe extracorporeal volume (EV) to maintain during treatment

1. Determine safe extracorporeal volume (EV) to maintain during treatment; suggested maximum EV is 15% total blood volume for adults and 10% for pediatric patients

  A. Pediatric patients

    (1) calculate pediatric blood and plasma volumes

    (2) include volume of ancillary devices to calculate total extracorporeal blood volume (e.g., blood warmer, cascade columns)

    (3) consider blood prime if patient size or condition warrants

2. Determine plasma volume and incorporate into treatment plan

3. Develop treatment plan

Patient Teaching

Before teaching begins, consider health literacy and individualize the approach by considering patient's cultural and health beliefs, preferences, and wishes

1. Explain reason for assessment

2. Describe how assessment parameters influence the treatment plan

References

Counts, C. (Ed.). (2008). *Core curriculum for nephrology nurses* (5th ed., p. 288). Pitman, NJ: American Nephrology Nurses' Association.

Kauffman, J., Myers, L., Rohe, R., & Axley, B. (2009). Clinical application: CQI aspects of the Therapeutic Apheresis Program. In B. Axley & K. Robbins (Eds.), *Applying continuous quality improvement in clinical practice* (2nd ed., pp. 125-130). Pitman, NJ: American Nephrology Nurses' Association.

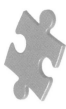

Equipment Assessment

Patient Outcome

The patient will receive a safe and effective treatment.

Nursing Care

Assessment

1. Prior to treatment initiation, the nurse will assess equipment and supplies, including
   A. Availability of emergency equipment and medications
      (1) for pediatrics: pediatric-specific equipment
      (2) for pediatrics: emergency medication calculated for weight or body surface area (BSA)
   B. Selection of appropriate equipment according to type of prescribed procedure (e.g., centrifuge, filter, column, or cascade)
   C. Equipment in proper working order and maintained according to manufacturer's recommendations
   D. Sterility and integrity of blood tubing, centrifuge bowl, plasma filter, adsorption column, or cartridge
   E. Sterility, prescription, and proper storage of replacement fluids
   F. Proper functioning of alarms, including air detector, red blood cell (RBC) spillover, blood leak, and pressure alarm limits if used
   G. Proper blood pump occlusion
   H. System is air-free after priming

Intervention

1. Make modifications based on equipment assessment prior to initiating treatment
2. Prime the extracorporeal circuit to remove all air, packing agent, or ethylene oxide sterilant according to established protocols

Reference

Counts, C. (Ed.). (2008). *Core curriculum for nephrology nurses* (5th ed., p. 288). Pitman, NJ: American Nephrology Nurses' Association.

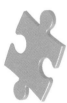

Initiation of Treatment

Patient Outcome

The patient will be free from complications related to the initiation of the procedure.

Nursing Care

Assessment

1. Inspect access site
2. Reassess vital signs prior to initiating therapy
3. Determine estimated plasma volume (EPV) (Calculate volume for pediatric patient)

Initiation of Treatment

4. Review prescription
   A. Exchange volume
   B. Anticoagulation
   C. Replacement fluid
   D. Calcium supplementation
   E. Blood prime for pediatric patients if indicated
5. Ensure that an efficient cycle time of blood products is achieved. Ensure that appropriate units of RBCs for erythrocytapheresis are available, ABO compatible and hemoglobin S negative, crossmatched, and screened for antibodies
6. Determine that appropriate informed consents are obtained
7. Verify appropriate matching of blood products used as replacement solutions according to institutional protocols

Intervention

1. Prepare vascular access for the initiation of the treatment according to established protocol
   A. Catheter prepared using aseptic technique
   B. Permanent vascular access for maintenance (i.e., AV fistula/graft)
      (1) return needle in direction of blood flow
      (2) needles at least 2 inches apart to prevent recirculation
      (3) needles 1.5 inches away from anastamosis
      (4) avoid aneurysms
      (5) 17-gauge arteriovenous fistula needles to prevent posttreatment bleeding
2. Collect blood specimens as ordered
3. Administer anticoagulation
4. Administer pretreatment medications as ordered
5. Connect access to the extracorporeal circuit
6. Secure connections between the patient and the extracorporeal circuit
7. Monitor integrity of extracorporeal circuit
8. Activate alarms and set limits

Reference

Kauffman, J., Myers, L., Rohe, R., & Axley, B. (2009). Clinical application: CQI aspects of the Therapeutic Apheresis Program. In B. Axley & K. Robbins (Eds.), *Applying continuous quality improvement in clinical practice* (2nd ed., pp. 125-130). Pitman, NJ: American Nephrology Nurses' Association.

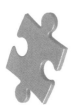

Anticoagulation

Patient Outcome

The patient will be free of complications of anticoagulation therapy.

Nursing Care

Assessment

1. Elicit history of injuries, surgical procedures, bleeding, and bruising
2. Review anticoagulation regimen from previous treatments
3. Review medication history, noting pharmacologic agents affecting anticoagulation

Anticoagulation

4. Assess for ecchymoses, hematomas, or other injuries
5. Review previous calcium levels, hemoglobin or hematocrit, prothrombin time (PT), international normalized ratio (INR), platelet count, and fibrinogen level
6. Review laboratory reports and history for evidence of heparin-induced thrombocytopenia (HIT)

Intervention

1. Monitor clotting times according to established protocol
2. Adjust anticoagulation regimen based on
   A. Established protocols
   B. Anticoagulation studies
   C. Patient condition
   D. Patency of extracorporeal circuit
   E. Response to previous anticoagulation
   F. When using citrate as the anticoagulant, monitor ionized calcium pretreatment and posttreatment to adjust IV calcium infusion rate and total dose
3. Individualize therapy for pediatric patients (e.g., citrate and heparin combination or increasing anticoagulant/blood ratio)
4. Observe for and treat complications
   A. Citrate
      (1) hypocalcemia
         a. clinical signs and symptoms
            [1] paresthesias
            [2] muscle cramps
            [3] muscle weakness
            [4] nausea or vomiting
            [5] malaise
            [6] hypotension
         b. in pediatric patients, observe for
            [1] restlessness
            [2] hyperactivity
            [3] listlessness
            [4] pallor
         c. changes in ionized calcium, electrolytes
         d. monitor serial blood levels based on nursing assessment
         e. arrhythmias
         f. assess for Chvostek and Trousseau signs
      (2) metabolic alkalosis
         a. clinical signs and symptoms
            [1] apathy
            [2] confusion
            [3] cardiac arrhythmias
            [4] neuromuscular irritability
            [5] depressed respirations
         b. changes in serum potassium, electrolytes, and arterial blood gases
      (3) hypernatremia
         a. irritability
         b. seizures
         c. muscle spasticity
         d. nausea and vomiting
         e. thirst
         f. labored respirations

Individualize therapy for pediatric patients

Anticoagulation

     g. decreased level of consciousness

     h. in pediatric patients, observe for

        [1] restlessness

        [2] hyperactivity

        [3] listlessness

        [4] pallor

        [5] serum sodium, other electrolytes

B. Heparin

  (1) bleeding or bruising

     a. around access site or other IV catheters

     b. oral cavity

     c. wounds

  (2) PTT and platelet count

  (3) clotting in extracorporeal circuit secondary to removal of protein-bound heparin

  (4) heparin rebound effect following treatment

C. Chilling

Patient Teaching

Before teaching begins, consider health literacy and individualize the approach by considering patient's cultural and health beliefs, preferences, and wishes

1. Signs, symptoms, and conditions to report
   A. Complications of anticoagulation therapy
   B. Signs and symptoms of hypocalcemia
      (1) metabolic alkalosis
      (2) hypernatremia
   C. Fatigue or weakness
2. Activity and precautions posttreatment

Reference

Kauffman, J., Myers, L., Rohe, R., & Axley, B. (2009). Clinical application: CQI aspects of the Therapeutic Apheresis Program. In B. Axley & K. Robbins (Eds.), *Applying continuous quality improvement in clinical practice* (2nd ed., pp. 125-130). Pitman, NJ: American Nephrology Nurses' Association.

Intratherapy Monitoring

Patient Outcome

The patient will receive a safe and effective treatment.

Nursing Care

Assessment

1. Patient
   A. Vital signs per protocol
      (1) monitor and document every 15-30 minutes or as necessary
      (2) cardiac monitoring should accompany any TPE treatment using intravenous citrate anticoagulation
   B. Blood product administration with documentation as required by institutional protocols

Intratherapy Monitoring

    C. Patient's condition
    D. Cardiac monitoring per protocol with attention to arrhythmias related to
        (1) electrolyte imbalance
        (2) cardiac irritation due to central lines
        (3) hemodynamic changes
        (4) patient's underlying condition
    E. Volume status by monitoring
        (1) intake, including anticoagulant volume, and output during treatment
        (2) hemodynamic changes
        (3) maintenance of extracorporeal volume within maximum limits based on patient assessment
    F. Response to blood product administration
        (1) appropriate warming of blood products
        (2) signs and symptoms of transfusion reaction
        (3) clotting abnormalities (PT, PTT, INR, fibrinogen, platelets)
    G. Effects of removal of highly protein-bound medications
        (1) hemodynamic changes
        (2) electrocardiogram (EKG) changes from baseline
        (3) physical changes
        (4) clotting
    H. Evidence of bleeding due to excessive anticoagulation or removal of clotting proteins
    I. Changes in baseline physical parameters, especially
        (1) respiratory changes
        (2) cardiac changes
        (3) neurologic changes
        (4) systems affected by underlying disease
    J. Vascular access function
        (1) ability to obtain desired blood flow rate
        (2) venous resistance
    K. Patient's subjective response to treatment
2. Treatment delivery system
    A. Integrity of extracorporeal circuit
    B. Anticoagulant delivery and effectiveness
    C. RBC spillover into plasma if applicable
    D. Pressure monitor readings
    E. Activation of alarms, alarm limits, and conditions

Implement age-appropriate emergency procedures according to patient's response to treatment

Intervention

1. Modify treatment plan based on assessment findings and in collaboration with health care team members
2. Administer medications, blood products, replacement fluids, and other treatments as ordered or per protocol
3. Implement treatment for blood product reaction, following established protocol as needed
4. Notify physician or advanced practice nurse of significant changes in patient's condition
5. Implement age-appropriate emergency procedures according to patient's response to treatment

Intratherapy Monitoring

Patient Teaching

Before teaching begins, consider health literacy and individualize the approach by considering patient's cultural and health beliefs, preferences, and wishes

1. Teach patient appropriate symptoms to report related to
   A. Blood product reaction
   B. Hypocalcemia
   C. Hypotension
   D. Chest pain
   E. Underlying disease process
2. Assist patient in identifying and implementing techniques to limit or manage adverse responses to treatment

Reference

Counts, C. (Ed.). (2008). *Core curriculum for nephrology nurses* (5th ed., p. 290). Pitman, NJ: American Nephrology Nurses' Association.

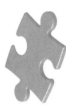

Fluid Management

Patient Outcome

The patient will maintain fluid volume status within established parameters.

Nursing Care

Assessment

1. Assess patient's
   A. Weight
   B. Blood pressure, sitting and standing
   C. Apical and peripheral pulses
   D. Central venous pressure (CVP) pulmonary artery wedge pressure (PAWP), if available
   E. Heart sounds
   F. Respiratory rate and breath sounds
   G. Presence or absence of edema
   H. Presence or absence of JVD
   I. Intake and output, fluid status
   J. Medications that influence volume status or hemodynamic parameters
   K. Disease-specific findings
   L. Laboratory and diagnostic test results

Intervention

1. Administer type and amount of replacement fluid as prescribed based on patient assessment
   A. Crystalloid solutions
   B. Colloid solutions
   C. Fresh frozen plasma or other blood products
2. Monitor volume of plasma removed and of replacement fluid administered
3. Monitor total intake and output
4. Monitor vital signs
5. Monitor for reactions to blood product

Fluid Management

Patient Teaching

Before teaching begins, consider health literacy and individualize the approach by considering patient's cultural and health beliefs, preferences, and wishes

1. Teach patient signs and symptoms of hypovolemia, hypotension, and fluid overload, and findings to report
2. Teach patient signs and symptoms of reaction to blood products and what to report

Reference

Kauffman, J., Myers, L., Rohe, R., & Axley, B. (2009). Clinical application: CQI aspects of the Therapeutic Apheresis Program. In B. Axley & K. Robbins (Eds.), *Applying continuous quality improvement in clinical practice* (2nd ed., pp. 125-130). Pitman, NJ: American Nephrology Nurses' Association.

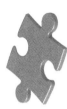

Acid/Base and Electrolyte Balance

Patient Outcome

The patient will maintain serum electrolytes and pH within safe parameters.

Nursing Care

Assessment

1. Assess for citrate-related complications (see Anticoagulation)
2. Review laboratory results and assess for clinical signs and symptoms of depletion of other substances contained in plasma that may occur when levels are low at the start of treatment
   A. Sodium
   B. Potassium
   C. Magnesium
   D. Phosphorous
   E. Calcium
   F. Bicarbonate

Intervention

1. Consult with physician regarding appropriate treatment of electrolyte or acid/base abnormalities and administer any medications or other treatments as prescribed
2. Avoid or treat excess citrate administration according to established protocol
   A. Slow blood flow rate
   B. Decrease amount of citrate
   C. Give supplemental calcium as ordered

Patient Teaching

1. Explain reasons for
   A. Possible hypocalcemia
   B. Other abnormalities that may occur
2. Teach patient to report signs and symptoms of
   A. Hypocalcemia
   B. Other electrolyte or acid/base abnormalities that may be expected based on pretreatment assessment findings

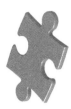

Complications

Common complications include blood leak, air embolus, and hemolysis.

BLOOD LEAK

Patient Outcome

The patient will be free of complications associated with blood leak.

Nursing Care

Assessment

1. Assess integrity of the extracorporeal circuit and delivery system alarms
2. Observe extracorporeal system for blood leaks
3. Observe color of plasma during initiation and throughout treatment for evidence of red blood cell contamination

Intervention

1. Correct any identified extracorporeal system problem or hazard that could lead to blood leak
   A. Loose connections
   B. Cracked bowl
   C. Improper loading of blood tubing
   D. Cracked tubing
   E. Filter or membrane damage
2. Use appropriate emergency interventions per established protocol if blood leak is suspected
   A. Stop procedure
   B. Assess vital signs
   C. Determine cause
   D. Observe patient for signs of hypovolemia and hypoxia and treat per established protocol
   E. Consult physician as needed
   F. Restart procedure

Patient Teaching

Before teaching begins, consider health literacy and individualize the approach by considering patient's cultural and health beliefs, preferences, and wishes

1. Teach patient signs and symptoms of hypotension and hypoxia
2. Explain emergency procedures

AIR EMBOLUS

Patient Outcome

The patient will be free of complications associated with air embolus.

Nursing Care

Assessment

1. Assess integrity of extracorporeal circuit and delivery system alarms, including vascular access
2. Engage air detect/line clamp device
3. Determine that the system is air-free after priming
4. Assess patient's vital signs, level of consciousness, and respiratory function per protocol

Intervention

1. Correct any identified extracorporeal system problem or hazard that could lead to an air embolus which includes, but is not limited to
   A. Loose connections or leaks
   B. Disengaged, disarmed, or nonfunctioning air detect/line clamp device
   C. Empty intravenous (IV) bags, blood bags, or infusion syringes
   D. Use of air-vented IV bottles
   E. Air in the extracorporeal circuit
   F. Inappropriate blood pump speed for access
2. Use appropriate connection techniques when using central venous catheters
3. Follow appropriate emergency interventions to include
   A. Stop treatment and clamp blood lines
   B. Position patient on left side with head lower than chest (modified Trendelenburg)
   C. Administer oxygen per established protocol
   D. Assess vital signs and level of consciousness
   E. Monitor cardiac status
   F. Assess and correct possible causes
   G. Notify physician
4. Use CQI process: identify areas of improvement, monitor changes, measure outcomes, and provide solutions to challenges

Patient Teaching

Before teaching begins, consider health literacy and individualize the approach by considering patient's cultural and health beliefs, preferences, and wishes

1. Review causes and prevention of air embolus
2. Teach patient symptoms to report to nurse or other health care team members
3. Explain emergency procedures

Reference

Kauffman, J., Myers, L., Rohe, R., & Axley, B. (2009). Clinical Application: CQI aspects of the Therapeutic Apheresis Program. In B. Axley & K. Robbins (Eds.), *Applying continuous quality improvement in clinical practice* (2nd ed., pp. 125-130). Pitman, NJ: American Nephrology Nurses' Association.

Determine that the system is air-free after priming

HEMOLYSIS

Patient Outcome

The patient will be free of hemolysis associated with treatment.

Nursing Care

Assessment

1. Assess integrity of the extracorporeal circuit and delivery system alarms
2. Determine whether hemolysis is likely related to disease process
3. Determine the rate of fluid removal
4. Assess color of plasma at initiation and throughout treatment
5. Assess response to treatment
6. Assess replacement solution administration
   A. Concentrated albumin volume is diluted with appropriate amount of 0.9% sodium chloride
   B. Dilution with other IV solutions (such as sterile water) creates a hypo-osmolar solution and results in hemolysis of red blood cells

Intervention

1. Monitor patient's vital signs and general status, equipment alarms, and rate of fluid removal throughout the treatment
2. If hemolysis is disease-related and expected, continue treatment
3. If treatment-related hemolysis is suspected, pause treatment and determine cause
4. If treatment-related hemolysis is determined, follow established protocol for emergency care, which may include
   A. Stop the plasma exchange, and do not return blood from extracorporeal circuit
   B. Check patient's vital signs
   C. Administer oxygen if indicated
   D. Notify the physician
   E. Send blood to lab to check for hemolysis
   F. Save circuit for analysis
   G. Administer intravenous (IV) fluids or blood transfusion according to established protocol
   H. Identify cause of hemolysis
   I. Observe patient for signs of hyperkalemia and hypoxia
   J. Restart treatment as appropriate

Patient Teaching

Before teaching begins, consider health literacy and individualize the approach by considering patient's cultural and health beliefs, preferences, and wishes

1. Teach patient to report
   A. Shortness of breath
   B. Chest pain
   C. Burning at access site
   D. Restlessness
   E. Generalized pain
2. Explain emergency procedures

Determine whether hemolysis is likely related to disease process
———

Reference

Kauffman, J., Myers, L., Rohe, R., & Axley, B. (2009). Clinical Application: CQI aspects of the Therapeutic Apheresis Program. In B. Axley & K. Robbins (Eds.), *Applying continuous quality improvement in clinical practice* (2nd ed., pp. 125-130). Pitman, NJ: American Nephrology Nurses' Association.

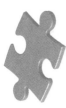

Termination of Treatment

Patient Outcome

The patient will be free from complications during termination of treatment and receive appropriate follow-up care.

Nursing Care

Assessment

1. Assess that treatment goals have been met
2. Appropriate type and volume of replacement fluids
3. Patient general sense of well-being

Intervention

1. Discontinue anticoagulation therapy according to the treatment prescription and as indicated by the nursing assessment
2. Follow established protocols to
   A. Return plasma and red blood cells in extracorporeal circuit to the patient
      (1) In cytapheresis, all components of the patient's blood are returned to the patient except for the targeted cells and any volume of plasma removed in conjunction with targeted cells
   B. Obtain any specimens ordered
   C. Disconnect from apheresis device
      (1) The patient's access and return lines must be disconnected prior to removing the disposable circuit set from the apheresis equipment; a failure to do so can result in excess fluid or air entering the patient's circulation
   D. Provide posttreatment access care per facility protocol
   E. Administer medications as ordered
   F. Dispose of plasma and treatment supplies
      (1) Use standard precautions for blood products
3. Reassess for changes from baseline and response to treatment
   A. Vital signs
   B. Body systems
   C. Patient's subjective response
4. Collaborate with other health care team members
   A. Document and communicate patient's response to treatment
   B. Provide treatment report to nurse responsible for posttreatment care
   C. Communicate patient status to primary consulting physician
   D. Arrange for follow-up care

Termination of Treatment

Patient Teaching

Before teaching begins, consider health literacy and individualize the approach by considering patient's cultural and health beliefs, preferences, and wishes

1. Signs and symptoms of posttreatment complications and appropriate interventions
   A. Hypotension
   B. Bleeding
   C. Hypocalcemia, hypernatremia, metabolic alkalosis, and other electrolyte imbalances as appropriate
   D. Hypervolemia
2. Routine care and precautions to maintain vascular access patency and prevent complications
3. Emergency contact numbers for health care team

References

American Society for Apheresis. (2010). Resources for apheresis professionals. American Society for Apheresis. Retrieved from http://apheresis.org/asfa_guidelines

Counts, C. (Ed.). (2008). *Core curriculum for nephrology nurses* (5th ed., p. 292). Pitman, NJ: American Nephrology Nurses' Association.

Kauffman, J., Myers, L., Rohe, R., & Axley, B. (2009). Clinical Application: CQI aspects of the Therapeutic Apheresis Program. In B. Axley & K. Robbins (Eds.), *Applying continuous quality improvement in clinical practice* (2nd ed., pp. 125-130). Pitman, NJ: American Nephrology Nurses' Association.

McKenna, R. (Coordinator). (2001). *Guidelines for education, training and competency in apheresis.* Sydney: Australian and New Zealand Apheresis Association. Retrieved from http://www.anzsbt.org.au/publications/documents/ANZAA_Apheresis_Education_Guidelines_Jun01.pdf

Passow, J., Pineda, A., & Burgstaler, E. (1984). Responsibilities of the registered nurse in the apheresis laboratory. *Journal of Clinical Apheresis, 2*(1), 1-6. Retrieved from http://www3.interscience.wiley.com/journal/113466992/abstract. DOI: 10.1002/jca.2920020104

Rosenthal, K. (2010). *Introduction to apheresis.* Retrieved from http://www.resourcenurse.com/about.html

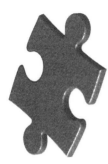

Continuous Renal Replacement Therapy

Continuous renal replacement therapy (CRRT) includes:

- Continuous venovenous hemofiltration (CVVH)
- Continuous venovenous hemodialysis (CVVHD)
- Continuous venovenous hemodiafiltration (CVVHDF)
- Slow low efficiency daily dialysis (SLEDD)
- Slow continuous ultrafiltration (SCUF)

I. Pretherapy

Pretreatment Assessment

Patient Outcome

The patient will receive safe and effective CRRT therapy and nursing care.

Nursing Care

Assessment

Pre-CRRT patient assessment includes a complete history of health and current diseases, current therapy and medications, and laboratory analyses as appropriate for patient condition. Family history, social history, allergies (both food products and drugs), and lifestyle activities may be obtained from the medical record.

1. Cardiac
   A. Blood pressure (baseline and current trends)
   B. Baseline electrocardiogram (ECG), pulse rate, rhythm
   C. Heart sounds: rubs or murmurs
   D. Apical and peripheral pulses
   E. Location and placement date of vascular access catheters; location and type of infusion lines and ports
   F. Hemodynamic parameters as applicable
      (1) central venous pressure (CVP)
      (2) pulmonary capillary wedge pressure (PCWP)
      (3) pulmonary artery diastolic pressure (PAD)
      (4) cardiac output (CO)
      (5) cardiac index (CI)
      (6) ejection fraction (EF)
      (7) stroke volume (SV)
   G. Jugular venous distention
   H. Cardiac medications
   I. Use of cardiac augmentation devices
      (1) intraaortic balloon pump (IABP)
      (2) type of temporary or permanent pacemaker (mode/rate)
      (3) ventricular assist device
      (4) extracorporeal membrane oxygenator (ECMO)
   J. Laboratory results, especially cardiac markers
   K. Diagnostic cardiac studies or operative reports if applicable
2. Pulmonary
   A. Breath sounds, respiratory effort, and rate
   B. Oxygenation status, arterial blood gases (ABG)
   C. Mixed venous oxygen saturation (SVO_2)
   D. Continuous oxygen saturation (oximeter SAO_2)

Pretreatment Assessment

E. Carbon dioxide partial pressure ($PaCO_2$)
F. Type of oxygen delivery system
G. Mechanical ventilation parameters if applicable
  (1) percent inspired oxygen (FIO_2)
  (2) tidal volume (TV) (delivered vs. received)
  (3) positive end expiratory pressure (PEEP)
  (4) continuous positive airway pressure (CPAP)
  (5) ventilation mode
    a. volume modes
      [1] controlled ventilation (CV)
      [2] controlled mandatory ventilation (CMV)
      [3] assist/controlled (AC)
      [4] intermittent (IMV) and synchronized intermittent mandatory ventilation (SIMV)
    b. pressure modes
      [1] pressure support ventilation (PSV)
      [2] pressure controlled/inverse ratio ventilation (PC/IRV)
  (6) extracorporeal membrane oxygenator (ECMO) or extracorporeal carbon dioxide removal (ECCOR)
  (7) high frequency oscillation ventilation (HFOV)
H. Arterial blood gas results
I. Diagnostic radiographic reports if applicable
J. Bronchoscopy reports if applicable

Monitor electrolyte components of the nutritional regimen

3. Neuromuscular
A. Mental status and trend of changes
B. Orientation to person, time, place, and purpose
C. Ability to communicate
D. Intracranial pressure (ICP) if monitored
E. Function of cranial nerves, including pupillary reactions
F. Tremors or asterixis of extremities
G. Bilateral deep tendon reflexes
H. Bilateral muscle strength and hand grasp
I. Ability to ambulate, change position, sit up
J. Sedatives, muscle relaxants, paralytic agents
K. History of seizure activity, type, duration, current meds

4. Gastrointestinal
A. Bowel sounds in all quadrants
B. Bowel pattern
  (1) normal
  (2) diarrhea
    a. infection control issues
  (3) no bowel movements
C. Nutritional considerations
  (1) Current calorie count and caloric requirements
  (2) Monitor electrolyte components of the nutritional regimen
    a. oral
    b. tube feeding
    b. parenteral
  (3) History of diabetes
    a. glucose management issues
    b. medications
    c. laboratory tests including liver function tests

Pretreatment Assessment

D. Bleeding
  (1) hematemesis
  (2) bloody nasogastric (NG) aspirate
  (3) melena and/or frank bleeding
E. Diagnostic radiographic reports if applicable
F. Diagnostic endoscopy or surgical reports if applicable

5. Renal
  A. Etiology of kidney failure
  B. Volume status
    (1) One of the most significant factors in caring for patients on CRRT is the basic principle of having an accurate intake and output
    (2) Standardizing the way(s) that care providers account for (add-up) intake and output and output (ultrafiltrate) could significantly improve the management of fluid and electrolyte balance in the CRRT patient
  C. Types and rates of fluids being administered (intake)
    (1) IV intake
    (2) enteral intake
    (3) TPN intake
    (4) oral if applicable
    (5) blood and blood components/products
  D. Types and amounts of fluid output
    (1) urine volume and output pattern
    (2) chest tube drainage
    (3) nasogastric drainage
    (4) wound drainage
    (5) stool
    (6) insensible losses
  E. Weight (current and preadmission)
  F. Edema
    (1) facial
    (2) extremity
    (3) abdominal (girth measurements)
    (4) dependent (sacral)
  G. Mucous membranes
  H. Laboratory results, including chemistries and ionized calcium
  I. Diagnostic renal studies
    (1) calculated or measured glomerular filtration rate (GFR)
    (2) radiographic reports
  J. Assess for history of underlying chronic kidney dysfunction (CKD)

6. Dermatologic
  A. Skin integrity, temperature, color, turgor
  B. Hematomas, induration, erythema
  C. Skin ulcerations, rashes, ecchymoses
  D. Presence and patency of indwelling intravenous, intra-arterial catheters, or central lines
  E. Presence and condition of drains, tubes, dressings
  F. Presence and stage of healing of surgical or trauma wounds

7. Hematologic and immunologic
  A. Presence of infection including but not limited to
    (1) human immunodeficiency virus (HIV)

> One of the most significant factors in caring for patients on CRRT is the basic principle of having an accurate intake and output

(2) hepatitis

    (3) methicillin-resistant *Staphylococcus aureus* (MRSA)

    (4) vancomycin-resistant *Enterococcus* (VRE)

    (5) *Clostridium difficile* (*C. diff*)

  B. Presence of fever or subnormal temperature

  C. Current antibiotics

    (1) Review of therapeutic levels

  D. Laboratory tests, including complete blood count, platelets prothrombin time (PT), and partial prothrombin time (PTT)

  E. Culture and sensitivity reports

8. Psychosocial

  A. Patient and family understanding of current illness

  B. Support systems available

  C. Religious affiliation or preference

  D. Patient and family's past effective coping mechanisms

Intervention

1. Develop plan of care in keeping with assessment findings
2. Collaborate with critical care team to integrate CRRT into the patient's plan of care
3. Develop and communicate plan for reassessment and evaluation
4. Monitor patient's response to CRRT therapy hourly and as needed

Teaching for Critical Care Nurses

It is assumed that the critical care nurse caring for the patient with AKI on CRRT will need additional education

1. Assist critical care nurse in identifying the pathophysiologic patient responses and complications secondary to acute kidney failure and CRRT therapy
2. Discuss the etiology of patient's kidney failure
3. Explain the rationale for evaluating existing kidney function and preexisting or concurrent conditions

Patient and Family Teaching

Before teaching begins, consider health literacy and individualize the approach by considering patient's and family's cultural and health beliefs, preferences, and wishes

1. Explain the patient's clinical condition and the purpose of CRRT; specifically, why the treatment is being performed and the expected clinical outcomes
2. Describe the CRRT procedure, including risks, vascular access, anticipated length of treatment, and patient positioning
3. Review the process of initiating therapy, the need for monitoring, possible side effects, and complications
4. Encourage and respond to questions from the patient and family

Collaborate with critical care team to integrate CRRT into the patient's plan of care

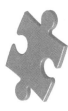

Preparation for Therapy Initiation

Patient Outcome

The patient will receive safe CRRT therapy.

Nursing Care

Assessment

1. Review and verify the CRRT treatment orders including
   A. Modality
   B. Vascular access
   C. Type of CRRT device or pump
   D. Type of hemofilter
   E. Blood pump speed
   F. Anticoagulant therapy
      (1) drug
      (2) dose
      (3) infusion rate
      (4) requisite lab tests
      (5) anticoagulant monitoring parameters
         a. PT/INR/PTT if using heparin
         b. calcium infusion rate and ionized calcium level if using intravenous citrate
   G. Replacement fluid (if used)
   H. Hourly ultrafiltration rate
   I. Hourly net fluid goals
   J. Dialysate solution and rate (if used)
   K. Frequency of blood pressure, vital signs, and hemodynamic measurements
   L. Laboratory results
      (1) electrolytes and parameters for repletion
      (2) critical values to be reported to nephrologist
2. Prepare and assess the CRRT system including
   A. Sterility of hemofilter and blood tubing as received from the manufacturer
   B. Prime CRRT circuit to remove all air, packing agent, and sterilant following manufacturer's instructions and established policy and procedures
   C. Replacement fluids are sterile and match prescription
   D. Dialysate is safe and matches prescription
      (1) dialysate and bicarbonate mixtures are within expiration date, clearly labeled with date and time of expiration
   E. Proper functioning of equipment including, but not limited to, blood pumps, pressure monitors, air alert detector, pressure and safety alarms
      (1) ensure that venous return line is placed in air detector since microbubbles may not be visible
      (2) equipment passes all tests in the test phase of setup and is within established industry standards
      (3) appropriate PM standards are met
      (4) RO water system is tested; chlorine/chloramines tested
   F. Assure access to a generator or emergency outlet for power
   G. Strategies in place for water supply and/or drain interruption

Preparation for Therapy Initiation

Teaching for Critical Care Nurses

It is assumed that the critical care nurse caring for the patient with AKI on CRRT will need additional education

1. Assist critical care nurse in identifying and understanding the prescribed CRRT modality
2. Teach critical care nurses appropriate emergency blood circuit rinseback procedure for the hemofilter design and CRRT technique to be used
3. Teach critical care nurses appropriate monitoring and problem-solving techniques related to CRRT equipment and processes
4. Instruct critical care nurses regarding appropriate safety precautions related to the use of CRRT equipment
5. Familiarize critical care nurses with equipment-specific monitoring of pressures and alarm systems
6. Teach critical care nurses how to test for chlorine every 4 hours or in accordance with hospital or corporate policy
7. Assure critical care nurse has access to the nephrology team for assistance with trouble shooting and problem-solving activities
8. Assure documentation of annual competencies regarding provision of CRRT therapy in accordance with Joint Commission standards and hospital or corporate policy

II. Intratherapy Considerations

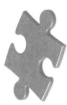

Initiation of Therapy

Patient Outcome

The patient will be free from complications related to initiation of the CRRT procedure.

Nursing Care

Assessment

1. Assess vascular access site(s)
2. Assess patient's vital signs immediately before connecting blood tubing to vascular access(es)
3. Check that pretreatment samples for laboratory tests have been obtained
4. Review patient condition and document that a verbal patient condition report was received from the primary nurse in accordance with applicable regulatory requirements and hospital and/or corporate policy.

Intervention

1. Identify patient according to institutional protocol
2. Position patient for comfort
3. Prepare vascular access(es) for initiation of therapy following established hospital and/or corporate protocols
4. Connect blood tubing to appropriate vascular access using sterile technique

Initiation of Therapy

5. If using a blood pump
   A. Check and set
      (1) blood flow
      (2) pressure monitor limits
      (3) air detector
   B. Start blood pump at half the ordered blood flow and/or in accordance with hospital/corporate policy, after assessing the patient's response, advance to the prescribed rate
6. Administer anticoagulant or initiate infusion, as applicable and in accordance with hospital/corporate policy
7. Administer dialysate countercurrent to blood flow at the prescribed rate if applicable
8. Begin ultrafiltration process as appropriate to type of CRRT equipment
9. Monitor and record the blood flow rate (BFR) and ultrafiltration flow rate (UFR) hourly, at a minimum. Document any changes as result of physician order and/or changes dictated by patient response
10. Secure the hemofilter and all line connections making sure to keep connections visible after initiation of treatment. Assure that appropriate disconnect prevention device is used in accordance with hospital/corporate policy
11. Monitor patient's response to initiation of therapy
    A. Changes in cardiac rate, rhythm, dysrhythmias
    B. Significant changes in blood pressure
    C. Physical changes such as dizziness, increased anxiety
12. Monitor for dialyzer or hemofilter reaction
    A. Hypotension and/or hypertension
    B. Pruritis
    C. Back pain
    D. Angioedema
    E. Changes in cardiac rate, rhythm, dysrhythmias
    F. Anaphylaxis

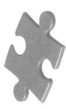

Intratherapy Monitoring

Patient Outcome

The patient will receive safe and effective CRRT treatment.

Nursing Care

Assessment

1. Monitor the following parameters throughout the CRRT therapy
   A. Patient
      (1) blood pressure, pulse, temperature
      (2) cardiac rhythm, rate, dysrhythmias
      (3) level of consciousness, mentation
      (4) intravascular and extravascular volume status
      (5) respiratory status and oxygenation
      (6) biochemical profile

Intratherapy Monitoring

       (7) coagulation and hematologic status

       (8) dialysis disequilibrium syndrome (DDS) (the possibility of DDS is low in CRRT)

         a. headache

         b. nausea and vomiting

         c. hypertension

         d. decreased sensorium

         e. convulsions

         f. coma

    B. CRRT system

       (1) security and patency of extracorporeal circuit

       (2) anticoagulant delivery and effectiveness

       (3) blood flow rate (BFR) and ultrafiltration rate (UFR)

       (4) arterial and venous pressure monitors

       (5) alarm limits and response

       (6) dialysate flow rate if applicable

       (7) replacement fluid rates if applicable

       (8) color and volume of ultrafiltrate

       (9) color and temperature of the blood circuit

Intervention

1. Administer fluids, medications, and blood products as prescribed or indicated based on patient's response

2. Obtain laboratory samples, report results, and modify therapy as ordered

3. Administer CRRT hourly replacement fluids based on prescribed net fluid loss or physician-planned CRRT regimen

4. In collaboration with the nephrology team, calculate the following upon request

    A. Sieving coefficient for a solute =

$$\frac{\text{ultrafiltrate concentration}}{\text{plasma concentration}}$$

    B. Convective clearance =

$$\frac{\text{ultrafiltration rate } \times \text{ ultrafiltrate concentration}}{\text{arterial concentration}}$$

    C. Diffusive clearance =

$$\frac{\text{dialysate flow rate } \times \text{ ultrafiltrate concentration}}{\text{arterial concentration}}$$

5. Keep hemofilter, blood tubing, and connections visible at all times. Stabilize extracorporeal circuit to avoid inadvertent tubing disconnections. Use appropriate disconnection prevention devices between the patient's access and the machine's blood line circuit

6. Maintain the hemofilter in an easily accessible position to allow for necessary nursing care

7. Discuss treatment modifications with physician based on patient response to therapy

8. Assist patient in position changes to prevent pressure points; if available use a therapeutic bed

Discuss treatment modifications with physician based on patient response to therapy

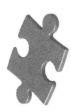

Anticoagulation

Patient Outcome

The patient will be free of complications related to anticoagulation therapy.

Nursing Care

Assessment

1. Assess patient's risk of bleeding from trauma, surgery, stress, or ulcerations (e.g., invasive line sites, surgical or trauma wounds, ecchymoses, hematomas)
2. Investigate patient's medical history related to bleeding disorders or events
3. Monitor patient for indications of bleeding
   A. Changes in coagulation indices and blood counts
   B. Decreased oxygenation
   C. Tachycardia and/or tachypnea
   D. Oozing of blood from catheters, drainage tubes, oral cavity
4. Assess patient's complete blood count and coagulation profile according to protocol
   A. Laboratory tests may include, but are not limited to
      (1) hemoglobin and hematocrit
      (2) platelet count
      (3) prothrombin time (PT)
      (4) partial prothrombin time (PPT)
      (5) activated clotting time (ACT)
      (6) fibrinogen level
      (7) ionized calcium level
5. Assess need for an alternative anticoagulation therapy range or alternative anticoagulant
6. Assess patency of CRRT circuit and hemofilter per institutional or corporate protocol
   A. Changes in arterial pressure
   B. Changes in venous pressure
   C. Changes in TMP
   D. Dark fibers in the hemofilter
   E. Separation of formed cells and serum in tubing (late sign)
   F. Decrease in hemofilter temperature (late sign)

Assess need for an alternative anticoagulation therapy range or alternative anticoagulant

Intervention

1. Administer anticoagulation as prescribed
2. Adjust anticoagulation administration based on patient's response and physician-ordered parameters
3. Perform interventions specific to the type of anticoagulation used
   A. Normal saline flushes
      (1) flush CRRT circuit with the ordered volume and frequency and as needed
      (2) add volume of flushes and/or prefilter fluids to hourly fluid intake
      (3) administer prefilter continous normal saline infusion via CRRT circuit as ordered
   B. Sodium heparin
      (1) administer loading dose prior to initiation of therapy

Anticoagulation

       (2) administer continuous infusion via CRRT circuit or central access as ordered

       (3) monitor dosing using ACT or activated partial thromboplastin time (aPTT)

       (4) monitor platelet levels to detect heparin-induced thrombocytopenia (HIT)

   C. Trisodium citrate

       (1) check composition of replacement fluid and dialysate

       (2) administer citrate via the CRRT circuit

       (3) infuse calcium chloride or calcium gluconate via central venous catheter

          a. calcium replacement is infused postcircuit or through central venous catheter to replace calcium losses as blood returns to patient

       (4) assess efficacy of anticoagulation by monitoring postfilter ACTs and/or ionized calcium

       (5) monitor serum sodium, bicarbonate, chloride, pH, and ionized calcium levels for acid/base and electrolyte imbalances

          a. monitor labs for alkalosis due to metabolism of citrate to bicarbonate

          b. monitor for hepatic inability to metabolize citrate

   D. Low molecular-weight heparin

       (1) administer loading dose prior to initiation of therapy

       (2) monitor Factor X levels

       (3) monitor platelet levels to detect heparin-induced thrombocytopenia (HIT)

   E. Hirudin

       (1) administer loading dose prior to initiation of therapy

       (2) monitor aPTT and ecarin levels

       (3) monitor for hirudin antibodies

   F. Argatroban

       (1) administer loading dose prior to initiation of therapy

       (2) monitor dosing using ACT or aPTT

4. If profuse bleeding occurs, discontinue CRRT immediately following established emergency termination procedure

5. If hemofilter or blood tubing clot, clamp blood lines, and disconnect CRRT system from vascular access(es) and discard

6. Maintain vascular access(es) according to established organizational protocol, pending reinitiation of CRRT

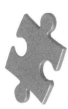

Fluid Management

Patient Outcome

The patient will achieve and maintain fluid volume balance within planned or anticipated goals.

Nursing Care

Assessment

1. Review pretherapy fluid status
2. Assess patient's response to the prescribed fluid management goals
3. Assess fluid losses and gains from all sources
4. Assess for peripheral, periorbital, facial, and sacral edema; changes in abdominal girth
5. Assess mucous membranes and skin turgor

Fluid Management

6. Assess breath sounds and oxygenation status
7. Assess heart sounds for gallop, rub, muffle, S3, or jugular venous distention
8. When available, assess central venous pressure
9. Assess laboratory and diagnostic test results

Intervention

1. Discuss hourly ultrafiltration rate (UFR) and desired hourly fluid balance with nephrology and critical care professionals
2. Alter fluid replacement as prescribed
3. Administer replacement and/or dialysate fluids as prescribed to achieve the planned fluid balance
4. Concentrate all intravenous medications and maintenance fluids to minimize total intake
5. Discuss adjusting mechanical ventilator settings in response to patient's clinical course with nephrology and critical care professionals
6. Estimate insensible fluid losses from skin and lungs
7. Review CRRT fluid balance calculations and machine setting interventions for accuracy

Acid/Base and Electrolyte Balance

Patient Outcome

The patient will achieve and maintain acid/base and serum electrolyte balance.

Nursing Care

Assessment

1. Assess changes from pre-CRRT laboratory values for
   A. Sodium
   B. Potassium
   C. Calcium
   D. Chloride
   E. Magnesium
   F. Bicarbonate
   G. Phosphorus
   H. Albumin
   I. Blood pH
2. Assess for dysrhythmias associated with serum electrolyte imbalance
3. Assess electrolyte intake from all fluid sources
4. Assess fluid status as it relates to serum sodium and albumin levels
5. Assess changes in arterial blood gases (ABG)
6. Assess patient's condition for non-CRRT-related factors contributing to electrolyte imbalance
7. Assess for correct dialysate and/or replacement fluids being administered based on prescription for composition and rates

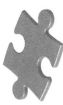

Acid/Base and Electrolyte Balance

Intervention

1. Collaborate with physician or advanced practice nurse for adjustments in fluids and medications
2. Adjust dialysate fluids, if used, to correct electrolyte imbalance
   A. Ensure fluids containing bicarbonate are not excessively warmed to prevent degradation of the component mixture
3. Administer intermittent electrolyte infusions for repletion as ordered
4. Administer parenteral nutrition or tube feedings with electrolytes to correct imbalances as ordered
5. Obtain 12-lead electrocardiogram (EKG) if indicated to interpret cardiac disturbances
6. Obtain laboratory tests as ordered or according to established protocols
7. In collaboration with physician, advanced practice nurse, or respiratory care provider, manipulate mechanical ventilator parameters to temporarily compensate for metabolic disturbances

Metabolic Stability

Patient Outcome

The patient will achieve and maintain metabolic stability during CRRT therapy.

Nursing Care

Assessment

1. Assess changes from pre-CRRT laboratory values for
   A. Creatinine
   B. Urea
   C. Potassium and other appropriate biochemical markers
2. Assess pharmacologic enteral and parenteral influences on any changes in patient's biochemical profile
3. Assess patient's underlying disease or condition for factors contributing to metabolic imbalances

Intervention

1. Submit laboratory samples; obtain and report results as appropriate and in accord with physician orders and/or established protocols
2. Calculate CRRT convective and/or diffusive solute clearance removal according to established protocol
3. Check clotting status of hemofilter in accordance with established protocols
4. Change CRRT system according to established policy
5. Collaborate with physician or advanced practice nurse to change CRRT modality as needed
6. Administer dialysate fluid countercurrent to blood flow through the hemofilter as prescribed

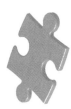

Nutrition

Patient Outcome

The patient will achieve and maintain adequate nutritional status.

Nursing Care

Assessment

1. Assess and compare current and preadmission weights
2. Assess nutritional intake of protein, calories, and lipids
3. Assess biochemical profile including albumin, prealbumin, and transferrin
4. Monitor blood glucose levels according to protocol
5. Assess bowel sounds and bowel patterns
6. Assess for muscle wasting, depleted adipose stores, and hair loss
7. Observe for changes in skin color, turgor, and temperature
8. Monitor for changes in soft tissue edema
9. Assess for loss of appetite

Intervention

1. Monitor daily weights
2. Administer nutritional supplement as prescribed
3. Estimate fluid loss from gastrointestinal disorders, diarrhea, vomiting, ostomy drainage
4. Administer insulin as prescribed
5. Collaborate with physician, advanced practice nurse, dietitian, and/or clinical pharmacist for nutrition support

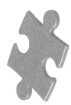

Complications

Complications include infection, hyperglycemia, hypothermia, and blood leak.

INFECTION

Patient Outcome

The patient will have no signs and symptoms of infection or sepsis.

Nursing Care

Assessment

1. Identify factors in patient's condition that may increase the risk of infection
2. Assess for signs and symptoms of infection including, but not limited to

A. Hyperthermia or hypothermia
B. Tachycardia
C. Hypotension, hemodynamic instability
D. Glucose intolerance
E. Areas of induration, warmth, swelling, tenderness, erythema, and purulent drainage
F. Inflammation at insertion site of intravenous or CRRT lines
3. Assess for changes in white blood count and differential
4. Identify risk of frequently clotted hemofilter

Intervention

1. Obtain samples for laboratory tests as ordered
2. Obtain cultures as ordered
3. In collaboration with physician or advanced practice nurse, monitor sites suspicious for infection
4. Administer antibiotics as prescribed with doses adjusted for the CRRT modality and clearance rates as appropriate
5. Perform dressing changes following established protocols
6. Monitor system regularly for signs of clotting

HYPERGLYCEMIA

Patient Outcome

The patient will maintain glycemic control during CRRT treatment.

Nursing Care

Assessment
1. Compare serial serum glucose levels with pre-CRRT values
2. Assess factors contributing to hyperglycemia
   A. Dialysate and intravenous solutions
   B. Sepsis
   C. Nutrition therapy
   D. Comorbid conditions

Intervention
1. Obtain serum glucose levels as ordered
2. Compare serum glucose levels with capillary blood glucose testing according to established protocol
3. Consult with dietitian for modifications in nutrition regimen
4. Collaborate with physician or advanced practice nurse to adjust concentration of glucose in the dialysate solution if possible and appropriate
5. Administer insulin as prescribed
6. Modify replacement fluid composition if indicated

HYPOTHERMIA

Patient Outcome

The patient will maintain body temperature within the prescribed range.

Nursing Care

Assessment

1. Note the desired therapeutic temperature
2. Compare serial temperatures
3. Assess for signs and symptoms of decreased body temperature
   A. Hemodynamic instability
   B. Chilling, shivering, or piloerection
   C. Skin pallor, coolness, cyanosis
4. Assess for factors contributing to a decrease in core temperature

Intervention

1. Provide the patient with extra blankets
2. Adjust CRRT machine's operational temperature in accord with physician order and recommended manufacturers limits
3. Use a warming blanket if indicated
   A. If using a warming blanket or extra blankets, maintain visibility of blood lines and connections to prevent accidental separation or exsanguination

BLOOD LEAK

Patient Outcome

The patient will not experience the complication of a CRRT circuit blood leak.

Nursing Care

Assessment

1. Assess color of ultrafiltrate after treatment initiation and routinely
2. Check ultrafiltrate for blood or hemoglobin per protocol
3. Assess changes in hemoglobin or hematocrit

Intervention

1. Assure CRRT machine passes all pretherapy alarm tests
2. Observe for ultrafiltrate color changes (amber to pink or red)
3. If ultrafiltrate offers evidence of a blood leak, follow unit protocol for treatment termination
4. Prepare for immediate system change

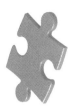

Minimal Interruption of Therapy

Patient Outcome

The patient will have minimal interruption in the delivery of CRRT therapy.

Nursing Care

Assessment

1. Evaluate actual hours of treatment per day as well as reasons for treatment interruptions

Intervention

1. Develop continuous quality improvement indicator trending tools to prevent interruptions
2. Use CRRT recirculation procedure when appropriate

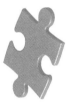

Termination of Therapy

Patient Outcome

The patient will be free from complications during termination of CRRT.

Nursing Care

Assessment

1. In collaboration with nephrology and critical care professionals, assess patient's need for further treatment
2. Assess CRRT circuit for clotting or leaks

Intervention

1. Standard disconnection
   A. Discontinue infusion of anticoagulant
   B. Discontinue dialysate flow
   C. Discontinue replacement fluids
   D. Monitor need for continued insulin infusion if used
   E. Return extracorporeal blood through the CRRT circuit using a normal saline flush according to manufacturer and unit specific protocol
   F. If using a catheter, flush with normal saline; cap with the prescribed solution according to protocol
   G Continue to monitor clinical and laboratory indicators
   H. Discard CRRT system as contaminated waste according to protocol
   I. The final hourly intake and output must be calculated and replacement fluid given as needed in accordance with physician order

2. Emergency termination for circuit leak, hemofilter rupture, clotting, circuit disconnection, dialyzer or circuit reaction, or to emergently move the patient
   A. Stop the blood pump
   B. Stop all pumps and infusions related to CRRT
   C. Clamp and disconnect blood lines; do not return blood to the patient
   D. If using a catheter, flush with normal saline; cap with the prescribed solution according to protocol (see Vascular Access section)
   E. Continue to monitor clinical and laboratory indicators
   F. Discard CRRT system as contaminated waste according to organizational environmental protocols

III. Posttherapy Considerations for Quality of Care

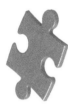

Posttreatment

In a collaborative team approach with the nephrology team and the ICU team, evaluate achievement of outcomes as listed above. Discuss changes and improvements that may further achievement of desired patient outcomes in the next treatment session.

Patient Outcome

The patient received safe and appropriate CRRT therapy.

Nursing Care

Assessment

1. Review the CRRT treatment, orders, and patient response (see Table 4.3)

Intervention

1. Implement changes and improvements as appropriate

Teaching for Critical Care Nurses

1. Review competencies as needed

Reference

Williams, H.F., Waack, T., & Axley, B. (2009). Clinical application: CQI in continuous renal replacement therapy. In B. Axley & K.C. Robbins (Eds.), *Applying continuous quality improvement in clinical practice* (2nd ed., pp. 133-139). Pitman, NJ: American Nephrology Nurses' Association.

Table 4.3
Elements of a CRRT Monitoring Tool

1. **General**
   A. Patient identification (e.g., name, medical record number, date of birth)
   B. Renal diagnosis
   C. Date treatment initiated
   D. CRRT modality
   E. Machine type and serial number
   F. Number of treatment days

2. **Vascular access**
   A. Insertion date
   B. Catheter type and size
   C. Catheter location
   D. Date of dressing change
   E. Site assessment
   F. Extremity assessment

3. **Circuit and filter**
   A. Filter type
   B. Circuit start date and time
   C. Circuit discontinued date and time
   D. Circuit/blood warmer temperature settings

4. **Dialysate and replacement fluids**
   A. Dialysate fluid
      (1) Composition
      (2) Date and time dialysate fluids changed
   B. Replacement IV fluids
      (1) Composition
      (2) Infusion site
      (3) Date and time IV bag(s) and infusion tubing changed

5. **Anticoagulation**
   A. Type of anticoagulant
   B. Ordered infusion rate
   C. Site of infusion
   D. Laboratory results

6. **Laboratory results monitoring**
   A. Serum chemistry
   B. Complete blood count with platelets
   C. Ionized calcium
   D. Prothrombin time and partial thromboplastin time
   E. Arterial blood gases

7. **System performance**
   A. Sieving coefficient
   B. Clearances

8. **Hourly assessment**
   A. Patient mental status
   B. Vital signs and hemodynamic data
      (1) temperature
      (2) pulse
      (3) blood pressure
      (4) mean arterial pressure
      (5) respiratory rate
      (6) central venous pressure
      (7) pulmonary capillary wedge pressure
      (8) pulmonary artery pressures
      (9) cardiac output or index
   C. Intake
   D. Output
   E. Desired fluid balance
   F. Replacement solution volume
   G. Ultrafiltrate volume
   H. Actual hourly fluid balance
   I. Fluid removal rate
   J. Blood flow rate
   K. Dialysate flow rate
   L. Anticoagulant infusion rate
   M. System pressures (e.g., arterial, venous, TMP)

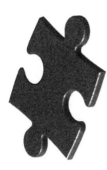

Kidney and Pancreas Transplantation

I. Deceased Donor

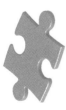

Approaching and Educating the Family

Patient Outcomes

The potential donor family will be provided with the option of organ and/or tissue donation in a sensitive manner after the patient has been determined to be medically eligible to donate.

The donor family will reach an informed and supported decision regarding organ and/or tissue donation that meets their emotional, religious, and cultural needs.

Deceased Donor – Approaching and Educating the Family

Nursing Care

Assessment

1. Recognize the criteria for brain death
2. Assess religious, cultural, and ethnic considerations of the family related to health care interventions, death, and organ and tissue donation
3. Determine the family's readiness to discuss options for organ and/or tissue donation
4. Understand the grieving process of families faced with the sudden death of a family member

Interventions/Family Education

1. Refer patients who have died or whose death is imminent to the local organ procurement organization (OPO) in a timely manner
2. Identify the legal next of kin who can discuss donation and give informed consent
3. Collaborate with the OPO to evaluate the suitability of the potential donor for organ and/or tissue donation
4. Collaborate with the OPO to provide the family with information regarding organ and/or tissue donation and answer any questions the family may have. Topics should include, but are not limited to
   A. Family's right to make an informed decision or to carry out the wishes of the patient
   B. Time limitations
   C. Options for organ and tissue donations
   D. Use of organs and tissue for transplant or research
   E. Allocation of organs and tissues
   F. Potential for nonuse of organs
   G. The donation process
      (1) guidelines for hemodynamic maintenance of the potential donor
      (2) surgical recovery of organs and tissues
      (3) medical examiner or coroner requirements
      (4) funeral or other arrangements
   H. Financial considerations
   I. Religious or cultural considerations
   J. Fear of mutilation
   K. Issues regarding anonymity
   L. Issues regarding patient dignity
5. Use culturally sensitive and ethnically appropriate educational materials or an interpreter if necessary
6. Provide adequate time and privacy for the family to make a decision
7. Support the family's decision to donate or not to donate

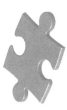

Physiologic Maintenance

Patient Outcome

The deceased donor will be physiologically maintained prior to organ recovery in an effort to maximize the number and quality of organs for transplantation.

Diseased Donor – Physiologic Maintenance

Nursing Care

Assessment

1. Organ procurement organization (OPO) will determine potential donor's eligibility based on established protocols and criteria, which may include, but are not limited to
   A. Verification of brain death
   B. Potential for organ donation after cardiac death
   C. Age
   D. Cause of death
   E. Previous medical and social history
   F. Absence of metastatic disease
   G. Absence of infection or transmissible disease
   H. Organ-specific suitability

Intervention

1. Call the local OPO for all imminent deaths
2. Obtain hemodynamic management guidelines from OPO
3. Assure adequate organ perfusion using established protocols including, but not limited to
   A. Maintain cardiopulmonary function including
      (1) blood pressure
      (2) heart rate
      (3) oxygenation using mechanical support
      (4) pharmacologic interventions as needed
   B. Prevent or treat infection
   C. Maintain electrolyte and acid base balance
   D. Maintain adequate hydration and treat diabetes insipidus as needed
   E. Maintain normothermia
4. Obtain samples for histocompatibility and serologic testing as directed by OPO

II. Living Donor

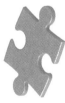

Education and Evaluation

Patient Outcome

The potential living donor will make an informed decision regarding organ donation and the evaluation process.

Nursing Care

Assessment

1. Identify potential donor's current level of knowledge
   A. Organ donation
   B. Histocompatibility testing
   C. Donor evaluation
   D. Risks and benefits of donation

**Living Donor –
Education and
Evaluation**

2. Obtain a complete nursing history that includes, but is not limited to
   A. Demographic data
   B. Occupation
   C. Past medical history
   D. Family medical history
   E. Current health status
   F. Current medications
   G. Current method of birth control
   H. Current health maintenance pattern
   I. Perception of general level of health
   J. Perception of outcome for the recipient
   K. Family dynamics and support systems
3. Perform a physical assessment

Intervention

1. Assist the potential donor in making an informed decision
2. Respect, support, and maintain confidentiality of the potential donor's decision
3. Prepare the potential donor for evaluation procedures
   A. Cross-matching and histocompatibility testing
   B. Laboratory testing
   C. Diagnostic procedures based on facility protocols
   D. Consultations

**Respect,
support, and
maintain
confidentiality
of the
potential
donor's
decision**

Patient Teaching

Before teaching begins, consider health literacy and individualize the approach by considering patient's cultural and health beliefs, preferences, and wishes

1. Implement a teaching plan that includes, but is not limited to
   A. Organ donation
   B. ABO compatibility
   C. Histocompatibility testing
   D. Donor evaluation
   E. Exclusionary donor candidate criteria
   F. Donor nephrectomy, open versus laparoscopic
   G. Potential benefits and risks of organ donation
   H. Convalescence
   I. Financial concerns and insurance issues
   J. Follow-up care
      (1) initial
      (2) long-term, including annual monitoring of creatinine, urinalysis, and blood pressure
2. Explain all tests and procedures
3. Explore the possibility of a nonfunctioning graft or kidney as well as the potential for recurrent disease in the kidney

Advanced Practice Nursing Care

(In addition to items outlined above)

Assessment

1. Assess the potential donor's risk factors related to kidney donation including family history, personal history, and existing medical conditions

**Living Donor –
Education and
Evaluation**

2. Assess the potential donor's risk factors for developing chronic kidney disease
3. Monitor potential donor's response to teaching regarding kidney donation

Intervention

1. Perform comprehensive health history and physical examination

Evaluation Studies

Patient Outcome

The potential donor will accurately complete diagnostic studies without complications.

Nursing Care

Assessment

1. Assess the potential donor's willingness to undergo multiple needle sticks required for obtaining blood samples and imaging studies
2. Assess the potential donor's ability and willingness to collect 24-hour urine collection at home if ordered
3. Obtain history of contrast allergy prior to imaging procedure
4. Postarteriogram
   A. Monitor vital signs, including temperature, at a frequency consistent with established protocol
   B. Assess for complications
      (1) Hematoma, swelling, or frank bleeding from puncture site
      (2) Absence of pedal pulse
      (3) Decreased urine output
   C. Assess level of postprocedure discomfort
7. Assess ability to undergo noninvasive procedures such as magnetic resonance imaging (MRI) (e.g., metal, claustrophobia)
8. Assess willingness and ability to complete all required tests as indicated (e.g., chest x-ray, electrocardiogram [EKG], Pap smear, mammogram)

**Assess
willingness
and ability to
complete all
required tests
as indicated**

Intervention

1. Postarteriogram
   A. Maintain bed rest with affected leg extended for an appropriate length of time
   B. Maintain adequate hydration to facilitate elimination of contrast
   C. Medicate with analgesic as ordered
   D. Apply pressure to arterial puncture site as indicated
2. For all contrast studies, maintain adequate hydration to facilitate elimination of contrast
3. For 24-hour collection, provide both verbal and written instruction and collection supplies

Patient Teaching

Before teaching begins, consider health literacy and individualize the approach by considering patient's cultural and health beliefs, preferences, and wishes

Living Donor – Evaluation Studies

1. For each procedure, explain purpose, complications, expected results, and frequency
2. Explain rationale for bed rest and adequate fluid intake after contrast studies
3. Teach signs and symptoms to report to the nurse
4. Inform the potential donor of the protocol that will be followed if any abnormal results are found

Advanced Practice Nursing Care

(In addition to items outlined above)

Assessment

1. Assess the potential donor's understanding of diagnostic studies

Intervention

1. Interpret results of laboratory tests and diagnostic imaging
2. Explain results to patient
3. Collaborate with the health care team in determining the eligibility of patient to donate

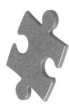

Perioperative Education and Discharge Planning

Patient Outcome

The potential living renal donor will demonstrate ability to participate in preoperative and postoperative regimens.

Nursing Care

Assessment

1. Assess current level of knowledge regarding the postoperative regimen
   A. Diet
   B. Medications
   C. Activity
   D. Signs and symptoms to report
   E. Expected length of hospital stay
   F. Postoperative home arrangements
   G. Follow-up appointments
   H. Timing of return to work
2. Evaluate readiness and ability to learn through assessment of
   A. Ability to concentrate
   B. Physical condition
   C. Psychological status
   D. Degree of motivation
   E. Developmental stage
   F. Literacy level
3. Identify potential barriers to learning that may include
   A. Physical condition
   B. Psychological status

Living Donor – Perioperative Education and Discharge Planning

    C. Environmental situation
    D. Cultural beliefs and practices
    E. Language
4. Evaluate effectiveness of teaching and learning by
    A. Verbal feedback
    B. Return demonstration
    C. Written test as appropriate

Intervention

1. Provide a comfortable and stress-free environment for preoperative teaching
2. Use teaching techniques and materials that are appropriate for the potential donor's developmental stage, disabilities, and cultural diversity
3. Include patient, family, spouse, or significant other in discharge planning
4. Refer to other resources for assistance in the learning process if necessary
5. Reinforce teaching using multiple teaching approaches if indicated
6. Arrange for home health care if required
7. Assure that follow-up appointments are scheduled
8. Confirm that prescriptions or medications are available

Patient Teaching

Before teaching begins, consider health literacy and individualize the approach by considering patient's cultural and health beliefs, preferences, and wishes

Provide a comfortable and stress-free environment for preoperative teaching

1. Implement a perioperative teaching plan that includes, but is not limited to
    A. Laboratory studies and x-rays
    B. Operating room environment
    C. Operating room attire
    D. Usual duration of surgical procedure
    E. Effects of preoperative medications and anesthesia
    F. Postoperative need for turning, coughing, deep-breathing, and ambulation
    G. Change in clinical setting postsurgery (e.g., medical intensive care unit, kidney transplant unit)
    H. Postoperative activity level
    I. NPO status and diet advancement
    J. Location and rationale for all tubes or drains including intravenous (IV) and urinary catheters
    K. Location of incision
    L. Level of pain to be expected and methods of pain control
    M. Postoperative nausea and methods to control it
    N. Postoperative constipation and methods to prevent or relieve
    O. Potential for temporary change in appearance related to fluid shifts
    P. Prophylactic measures for deep vein thrombosis
    Q. Potential emotional response to loss of body part
    R. Potential for nonfunctioning transplanted kidney in recipient or recurrent disease
2. Develop and implement a discharge teaching plan that includes, but is not limited to
    A. Heavy lifting limitations
    B. Operation of motor vehicle
    C. Exercise
    D. Sexual activity
    E. Medications, including over-the-counter medicines, to avoid, restrict, or use
    F. Diet and fluid management
    G. Care of operative site

Living Donor – Perioperative Education and Discharge Planning

H. Signs and symptoms to report to the primary care provider or transplant team
I. Date and time of follow-up appointment
J. Return to work

Advanced Practice Nursing Care

(In addition to items outlined above)

Assessment

1. Assess patient's understanding of the donation process
2. Reinforce previous teaching

Interventions

1. Coordinate discharge care

III. Recipient

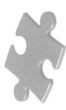

Education and Evaluation

Patient Outcomes

The patient will make an informed decision regarding transplantation.

The patient will participate in the pretransplant evaluation procedures.

Nursing Care

Assessment

1. Identify current level of knowledge related to the evaluation process, histocompatibility testing, transplantation, and current insurance plan
2. Assess pretransplant (current) adherence to treatment plan

Interventions

1. Involve support person/family in teaching process
2. Encourage verbalization of anxieties, fears, and questions
3. Refer questions to appropriate health care personnel
4. Assist the potential transplant candidate in making an informed decision
5. Respect, support, and maintain confidentiality of the patient's decision
6. Prepare the patient for evaluation procedures
    A. Cross-matching and histocompatibility testing
    B. Routine laboratory tests
    C. Diagnostic tests per established protocols
    D. Consultations
7. Administer immunizations as ordered

Patient Teaching

Before teaching begins, consider health literacy and individualize the approach by considering patient's cultural and health beliefs, preferences, and wishes

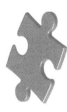

Recipient – Education and Evaluation

1. Implement a teaching plan that includes, but is not limited to
   A. Kidney transplantation
   B. Pancreas transplantation when appropriate
   C. Potential benefits and risks of transplantation
   D. Patient and family responsibilities pretransplant and posttransplant
   E. Deceased versus living (related or unrelated) renal donor transplantation
   F. Immunosuppressive therapy
   G. Histocompatibility testing
   H. Pretransplant evaluation
   I. Exclusion criteria for potential recipients
   J. Time on waiting list and protocols for patient selection when organ is available
   K. Surgical procedure including native nephrectomy when appropriate
   L. Convalescence
   M. Financial issues including costs of medications and self-monitoring equipment
   N. Follow-up care
   O. Importance of adherence to treatment plan
2. Explain all tests and procedures to the patient
3. Discuss with patient the possible emotional responses of family members or significant others to the request for evaluation as a potential organ donor
4. Refer to social worker to identify sources of social as well as financial support pretransplant and posttransplant

Perioperative Education and Discharge Planning

Patient Outcomes

The patient will participate in perioperative and discharge education.

The patient will demonstrate the ability to participate in and follow the posttransplant regimen both as an inpatient and postdischarge.

Nursing Care

Assessment

1. Assess current level of knowledge regarding posttransplant
   A. Diet
   B. Fluid intake
   C. Medications
   D. Activity including return to work or school
   E. Oral hygiene
   F. Infection
   G. Rejection
   H. Signs and symptoms to report
   I. Sexuality
   J. Postdischarge home arrangements
   K. Follow-up appointments

L. Insurance coverage for
  (1) medications
  (2) follow-up care with transplant center
  (3) primary care provider

Interventions

1. Include patient, family, spouse, or significant other in preoperative and discharge planning
2. Arrange for home health care if required
3. Assure that follow-up appointments are scheduled and patient is aware of appointment schedule
4. Confirm that prescriptions or discharge medications are available
5. Provide patient with materials to manage home care
   A. Medication list
   B. Essential phone numbers
   C. Written materials
   D. MedicAlert application
6. Initiate appropriate referrals

Patient Teaching

Before teaching begins, consider health literacy and individualize the approach by considering patient's cultural and health beliefs, preferences, and wishes

**Clarify issues
and concerns
regarding
expected
changes in
health status,
lifestyle, or
role function**

1. Preoperative education
   A. Implement a teaching plan that includes, but is not limited to
      (1) preoperative medications and anesthesia
      (2) usual duration of surgical procedure
      (3) postoperative need for turning, coughing, deep breathing, ambulation, incentive spirometer use
      (4) changes in clinical setting postsurgery (e.g., intensive care unit, kidney transplant unit)
      (5) postoperative activity levels
      (6) NPO status and diet advancement
      (7) location and rationale for tubes and drains
      (8) location of incision
      (9) amount of incisional pain to be expected
      (10) methods of pain control
      (11) immunosuppressive therapy
      (12) infection prophylaxis
      (13) early postoperative body changes related to surgical procedure and edema
      (14) expectations regarding patient's responsibility for
          a. self-administration of medications
          b. education while hospitalized
      (15) potential complications such as delayed graft function and the need for dialysis in the immediate postoperative period
      (16) postoperative surveillance tests
          a. ultrasound
          b. kidney biopsy
   B. Clarify issues and concerns regarding expected changes in health status, lifestyle, or role function
   C. Request that the social worker clarify insurance coverage for medications and follow-up care with transplant center and primary care physician
   D. Discuss options regarding pharmacies and outside laboratories to use after discharge

Recipient – Perioperative Education and Discharge Planning

2. Postoperative and discharge teaching
  A. Implement a teaching plan for the patient and family that includes, but is not limited to
    (1) medications
        a. types
        b. purpose
        c. dosage and frequency of administration
        d. route
        e. side effects and precautions
        f. drug interactions, including herbs and grapefruit
        g. over-the-counter medications to avoid, restrict, or use
        h. importance of reporting all medications ordered by other providers to the transplant team
        i. importance of immunosuppressant blood trough levels
        j. consult transplant team before using generic immunosuppressant medications
    (2) infection
        a. signs and symptoms to report
        b. health practices to reduce exposure to infectious agents, including immunizations and antibiotic prophylaxis for dental procedures
    (3) rejection
        a. probability and causes
        b. signs and symptoms to report
        c. monitoring of weight and temperature
        d. how to contact the nephrology and transplant teams
        e. management of acute and chronic rejection
        f. consequences of irreversible rejection
    (4) diet and fluid prescription
        a. components of a well-balanced diet
        b. fluid intake
        c. restrictions
        d. drug or food interactions
        e. measures for weight control
        f. effects of medications on appetite
    (5) home arrangements
        a. home therapy as indicated
        b. housekeeping and cleanliness
        c. child care
        d. activities of daily living
    (6) activities
        a. importance of a regular exercise program
        b. type and duration of activity restrictions
        c. return to work or school
    (7) sexuality
        a. physiologic changes
        b. emotional reactions
        c. contraception and safe sex practices
        d. pregnancy
        e. breast self-exam and PAP smears
        f. testicular self-exam and need for regular prostate exam
    (8) other health maintenance practices
        a. regular dental care
        b. smoking cessation
        c. moderate alcohol consumption

Implement a teaching plan for the patient and family

    d. good skin care
    e. importance of avoiding potentially hazardous environmental situations such as demolition and renovation projects
    f. avoiding contact with others who are ill with cold, flu, or infections
    g. annual physical exams
    h. continued need for up-to-date immunizations
    i. routine surveillance studies (e.g., mammogram, colonoscopy, prostate-specific antigen [PSA], bone mineral density scan)
  (9) follow-up care
    a. rationale for follow-up care
    b. scheduling visits
    c. blood and urine testing
    d. medication regimen
    e. self-monitoring
    f. maintenance of logs per unit protocol
    g. medication refill process
    h. phone numbers and procedures to use when patient has questions
    i. transportation to and from clinic or laboratory
    j. community resources

Advanced Practice Nursing Care

(In addition to items outlined above)

Assessment

1. Assess patient's understanding of transplant process
2. Reinforce previous teaching

Interventions

1. Coordinate discharge care

IV. Postoperative Care of Donors and Recipients

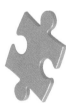

Pulmonary Care

Patient Outcome

The patient will maintain adequate respiratory function.

Nursing Care

Assessment

1. Assess respiratory status
   A. Breath sounds
   B. Rate
   C. Depth
   D. Drive or effort

Postoperative Care of Donors and Recipients – Pulmonary Care

E. Character and consistency of expectorated sputum

F. O_2 saturation

G. Arterial blood gas (ABG) results

2. Monitor vital signs at a frequency consistent with established protocol

3. Assess level of consciousness

4. Assess use of narcotics

Intervention

1. Administer oxygen as prescribed
2. Encourage patient to perform pulmonary toilet/hygiene
3. Provide chest physical therapy as necessary
4. Appropriate use of incentive spirometer
5. Administer analgesics as ordered to make coughing and deep-breathing more tolerable
6. Allow patient adequate time for rest between exercises to prevent fatigue
7. Assist patient to ambulate after surgery per established protocol
8. Have narcotic antagonist available and administer as ordered

Patient Teaching

Before teaching begins, consider health literacy and individualize the approach by considering patient's cultural and health beliefs, preferences, and wishes

1. Explain the importance of coughing and deep-breathing
2. Demonstrate "splinting" of incision during coughing to facilitate incisional comfort
3. Demonstrate appropriate technique to get out of bed

Advanced Practice Nursing Care

(In addition to items outlined above)

Assessment

1. Monitor the patient's response to the treatment plan
2. Interpret results of diagnostic testing

Intervention

1. Order and interpret additional diagnostic testing as the patient's condition warrants
2. Adjust medication regimen based on assessment of patient
3. Collaborate with other members of the health care team as needed

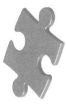

Fluid Management

Patient Outcome

The patient will achieve desired fluid volume status.

Nursing Care

Assessment

1. Systematically assess
    A. Cardiovascular function
        (1) heart sounds
        (2) blood pressure
        (3) pulse rate

Postoperative Care of Donors and Recipients – Fluid Management

        (4) cardiac rhythm
        (5) edema
        (6) central venous pressure (CVP) per established protocol
        (7) jugular vein distention (JVD)
        (8) vascular access
    B. Pulmonary function
        (1) respiratory rate
        (2) breath sounds
        (3) cough
        (4) dyspnea
    C. Gastrointestinal (GI) function
        (1) abdominal distention
        (2) bowel sounds
        (3) flatus
    D. Fluid balance
        (1) thirst
        (2) intake and output
        (3) urine output
    E. Skin turgor and mucous membranes
    F. Lab values
        (1) blood urea nitrogen (BUN) and serum creatinine
        (2) hemoglobin and hematocrit
        (3) electrolytes
2. Monitor daily weight gain or loss
3. Monitor output from drains

Encourage or assist with ambulation to mobilize edema

Intervention

1. Maintain accurate records of fluid intake and output
2. Maintain adequate fluid balance by administering fluid or diuretics as ordered
3. Encourage or assist with ambulation to mobilize edema
4. Protect edematous areas from injury or breakdown
5. Encourage oral fluid intake to prevent dehydration

Patient Teaching

Before teaching begins, consider health literacy and individualize the approach by considering patient's cultural and health beliefs, preferences, and wishes

1. Teach the patient and family how to measure and record intake and output
2. Explain reason for changes in fluid volume
3. Explain the rationale for adequate fluid intake or diuretics

Advanced Practice Nursing Care

(In addition to items outlined above)

Assessment

1. Assess the patient's volume status
2. Interpret diagnostic studies
3. Monitor response to the treatment regimen

Intervention

1. Adjust intravenous fluids and diuretics based on patient's response to treatment plan
2. Order additional diagnostic studies according to patient condition

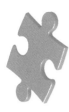

Bowel Function

Patient Outcome

The patient will establish a desired bowel elimination pattern.

Nursing Care

Assessment

1. Assess for presence of nausea, vomiting
2. Assess appetite
3. Assess patient's abdomen daily for pain and distention
4. Auscultate for bowel sounds and assess for passage of flatus
5. Assess the quantity and character of stool
6. Assess need for laxatives
7. Assess history of bowel patterns and use of drugs that alter gastrointestinal motility
8. Assess narcotic use
9. Assess mobility and activity level

Intervention

1. Administer antiemetics as ordered
2. Once flatus has been passed, advance diet as tolerated and ordered
3. Encourage adequate intake of fluid and fiber
4. Provide privacy and normal positioning for bowel movement
5. Consult renal dietitian if indicated
6. Administer laxatives or other elimination aids as ordered; evaluate effectiveness
7. Encourage or assist patient to ambulate
8. Consult with physician or advanced practice nurse to reinstitute motility drugs after ileus is resolved

Patient Teaching

Before teaching begins, consider health literacy and individualize the approach by considering patient's cultural and health beliefs, preferences, and wishes

1. Discuss the importance of activity and its relationship to bowel function
2. Counsel regarding adequate dietary intake
3. Teach the patient to report to the nurse any changes in color or consistency of stool
4. Explain the effects of narcotics and transplant medications on bowel function

Advanced Practice Nursing Care

(In addition to items outlined above)

Assessment

1. Assess patient's response to the treatment regimen

Interventions

1. Order antiemetics, laxatives, or other elimination aids as indicated by patient condition

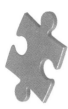

Urinary Tract Infection

Patient Outcome

The patient will maintain adequate urine output and void spontaneously.

Nursing Care

Assessment

1. Review preoperative assessment of anatomy and function of the urinary tract
2. Assess color, clarity, and quantity of urine
3. Assess fluid intake
4. Assess for distended bladder
5. Assess patency of urinary catheter if present
6. Assess for lower abdominal pain or burning
7. Assess recipient's wound for drainage; assess creatinine of copious drainage
8. Assess for bladder spasms
9. Assess patient's perception of ability to empty bladder
10. Assess use of narcotics
11. Assess for urine leak

Intervention

1. Maintain catheter patency per established protocol
2. Notify physician or advanced practice nurse of significant decrease in urine volume or change in color or clarity of urine
3. After catheter is removed, encourage patient to void frequently
4. Notify physician or advanced practice nurse if patient is unable to void spontaneously
5. Check postvoid residual volume in bladder per established protocol
6. Catheterize bladder as ordered
7. While catheter is in place, administer antispasmodics as ordered
8. When catheter is removed, administer medications to aid voiding as ordered

Patient Teaching

Before teaching begins, consider health literacy and individualize the approach by considering patient's cultural and health beliefs, preferences, and wishes

1. For the patient with a urinary catheter, explain catheter purpose and potential complications
2. Teach the patient how to measure urine output
3. Teach the patient signs and symptoms of urinary dysfunction to report
4. Teach good hygiene practices
5. Discuss measures to prevent urinary tract infection
6. Prepare patient for diagnostic studies to evaluate urinary function
7. Teach patient to self-catheterize as needed
8. For bladder-drained pancreas recipients, explain reason for more viscous and discolored urine

Postoperative Care of Donors and Recipients – Urinary Tract Infection

Advanced Practice Nursing Care

(In addition to items outlined above)

Assessment

1. Assess patient's response to the treatment regimen

Intervention

1. Order and interpret additional diagnostic studies as indicated by patient condition
2. Coordinate care with other members of the health care team

Operative Site Care

Patient Outcome

The patient will maintain an incision that is intact and free from complications.

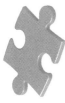

Nursing Care

Assessment

1. Assess incision for
    A. Evidence of bleeding
    B. Infection
    C. Drainage
    D. Impaired healing
    E. Swelling
    F. Blisters
2. Assess drains for patency, type, and quantity of drainage
3. Assess for abdominal pain related to leakage of blood, urine, or amylase (in pancreas transplant)

Intervention

1. Change dressings as needed
2. Maintain patency of drains, suction as ordered
3. Notify physician or advanced practice nurse if any significant change is noted
4. Protect operative site from injury
5. Make home care referral as needed

Patient Teaching

Before teaching begins, consider health literacy and individualize the approach by considering patient's cultural and health beliefs, preferences, and wishes

1. Discuss short-term and long-term activity limitations and body mechanics to protect wound and promote comfort
2. Teach patient and family care of wound
3. Teach signs and symptoms of wound infection and other related problems to report to the nurse

Postoperative Care of Donors and Recipients – Operative Site Care

Advanced Practice Nursing Care

(In addition to items outlined above)

Assessment

1. Assess operative wound for signs of infection and delayed healing

Intervention

1. Perform incision and drainage if signs of infected wound
2. Determine appropriate wound care based on depth, location, and type of wound
3. Order antibiotics as needed
4. Monitor response to prescribed regimen

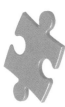

Comfort Management

Patient Outcome

The patient will achieve comfort postoperatively.

Nursing Care

Assessment

1. Identify patient's cultural and psychosocial response to pain
2. Assess preoperative use of analgesics and comfort measures
3. Monitor vital signs per established protocol
4. Assess objective and subjective evidence of pain
5. Assess location and severity of pain
6. Assess ability to perform activities of daily living
7. Assess effectiveness and side effects of analgesic medication and other pain-reducing measures

Intervention

1. Provide analgesics
    A. Patient-controlled analgesia
    B. Epidural analgesia
    C. Medicate as ordered
2. Provide analgesics prior to activity
3. Assist patient in the use of relaxation techniques
4. Assist patient to a position of comfort
5. Allow patient adequate time for sleep and rest between activities
6. Encourage patient to resume usual activity level and perform activities of daily living at an appropriate pace
7. Provide assistance as needed to ambulate and perform activities of daily living
8. Encourage diversional activities

Postoperative Care of Donors and Recipients – Comfort Management

Patient Teaching

Before teaching begins, consider health literacy and individualize the approach by considering patient's cultural and health beliefs, preferences, and wishes

1. Provide information regarding reason for pain or discomfort, expected duration, and measures for relief
2. Discuss side effects of narcotics
3. Explain how to ask for pain medication or how to use patient-controlled analgesia

Advanced Practice Nursing Care

(In addition to items outlined above)

Assessment

1. Assess patient's response to treatment regimen

Intervention

1. Adjust analgesic type and dosage based on patient response
2. Discuss adjunct treatments that may help with pain control
3. Monitor patient response to treatment

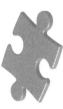

Allograft Dysfunction

Patient Outcome

The patient will demonstrate an understanding of allograft dysfunction and participate in its management.

Nursing Care

Assessment

1. Assess for evidence of allograft dysfunction
   A. Renal transplant
      (1) blood urea nitrogen (BUN), creatinine, electrolytes
      (2) intake and output; comparison with pretransplant urine output
      (3) weight
      (4) edema
      (5) respiratory status
   B. Pancreas transplant
      (1) blood glucose
      (2) serum amylase and lipase
      (3) urinary amylase
      (4) eosinophils (bladder-drained pancreas only)
2. Assess for evidence of prerenal or prepancreas causes of allograft dysfunction
   A. Hypovolemia, dehydration
   B. Hypotension, low cardiac output
   C. Bleeding
      (1) from incision or drain
      (2) abdominal pain caused by blood irritating surrounding tissues

Postoperative Care of Donors and Recipients – Allograft Dysfunction

        (3) diminished peripheral pulses

    D. Kidney only

        (1) use of angiotensin-converting enzyme (ACE) inhibitors or vasoconstrictive agents, including cyclosporine and tacrolimus

        (2) bruit over renal artery

        (3) sudden increase in blood pressure

        (4) hematuria (renal vein thrombosis)

3. Assess for evidence of postrenal/postpancreas causes of allograft dysfunction
   A. Urinary catheter patency or ability to empty bladder efficiently*
   B. Abnormal drainage from incision or drains
   C. Swelling or pain near allograft
   D. Urinary tract infection*

4. Assess for evidence of intra-organ causes of allograft dysfunction
   A. Duration of ischemia prior to transplantation
   B. Tenderness over graft
   C. Nonadherence to immunosuppressive regimen
   D. Temperature
   E. Hypersensitivity reactions
   F. Recent illness and activity
   G. Kidney only
      (1) proteinuria, hematuria
      (2) potential for recurrence of original renal disease
      (3) use of nephrotoxic contrast agents and drugs
      (4) medications that alter drug levels of immunosuppressive medications

5. Review results of diagnostic studies

6. Assess emotional status

7. Assess factors affecting adherence to medical regimen

8. After biopsy of transplanted organ, assess for
   A. Bleeding, swelling, hematoma, pain at biopsy site
   B. Peripheral pulses
   C. Hematuria*
   D. Ability to void*
   E. Vital signs
   F. New bruit over organ

Monitor for effectiveness and side effects or complications of immuno-suppressive therapy

Intervention

1. Notify physician or advanced practice nurse of significant changes
2. Irrigate catheter or catheterize bladder, as ordered
3. Obtain orders for fluids or diuretics and administer as ordered
4. Prepare patient for diagnostic procedures per established protocol
5. Administer immunosuppressive therapy, as ordered
6. Monitor for effectiveness and side effects or complications of immunosuppressive therapy
7. Provide emotional support
8. Request or initiate consultations and referrals as appropriate

Patient Teaching

Before teaching begins, consider health literacy and individualize the approach by considering patient's cultural and health beliefs, preferences, and wishes

1. Explain cause of graft dysfunction, its usual course, treatment, and long-term implications

Postoperative Care of Donors and Recipients – Allograft Dysfunction

2. Explain potential need for dialysis until kidney function is adequate
3. Teach importance of and reasons for adhering to fluid and diet prescriptions
4. Review medications
   A. Types
   B. Purpose
   C. Dose and route
   D. Implications of not taking medications as ordered
   E. Side effects, interactions, and precautions
5. Review signs and symptoms of complications to report to transplant or nephrology team
6. Teach patient importance of notifying transplant team immediately of change in insurance or financial status, especially as it pertains to coverage of outpatient medications

* Does not apply to enteric-drained pancreas transplant

Advanced Practice Nursing Care

(In addition to items outlined above)

Assessment

1. Assess patient for allograft dysfunction

Interventions

1. Order and interpret additional diagnostic studies as indicated by patient condition (e.g., ultrasound, biopsy, laboratory tests)
2. Adjust medications as needed
3. Monitor patient for response to treatment regimen

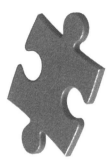

Palliative Care and End-of-Life Care

Palliative care is an approach that improves the quality of life of patients and their families facing the problems associated with life-threatening illness, through the prevention and relief of suffering by means of early identification and impeccable assessment and treatment of pain and other problems, physical, psychosocial, and spiritual (World Health Organization, 1998). Palliative care for patients with kidney disease includes physical, psychological, social, spiritual, and end-of-life care.

End-of-life (EOL) care is a subset of palliative care that includes hospice. Both palliative and hospice care focus on quality of life and comfort and supportive measures rather than curative interventions.

Patient Outcome

The patient and family will receive guidance with advance care planning and, if applicable, dialysis facility policies related to advance medical directive (AMD) and end-of-life care (EOL).

The patient will receive appropriate pain and symptom management, and psychosocial and spiritual support throughout the acute renal failure, chronic kidney disease, and dying experiences that include palliative and hospice care.

Nursing Care

Assessment

1. Review patient's preparedness for EOL by assessing knowledge of advance care planning and presence of documented decisions or verbalized wishes that include
   A. Living will
   B. Health care power of attorney or health care proxy
   C. Order for "Do not resuscitate" (DNR) or "Allow natural death" (AND)
   D. Specific circumstances that the patient feels would warrant reevaluation of treatment goals such as a terminal diagnosis, need for amputation, or frequent hospitalizations
2. Assess for
   A. Level and state of consciousness
   B. Level of mobility
   C. Circulation
   D. Appetite
   E. Hydration
   F. Quality of sleep
   G. Skin integrity
   H. Presence and degree of pain
   I. Capacity to make decisions
   J. Other physical signs and symptoms and the degree to which they cause patient suffering or discomfort including
      (1) shortness of breath

      (2) pruritis
      (3) restlessness
      (4) nausea and vomiting
      (5) constipation or diarrhea
      (6) feeling cold

K. Psychological and emotional status, including
      (1) problem-solving abilities
      (2) cognitive function
      (3) behavior
      (4) anxiety
      (5) depression
      (6) coping mechanisms
      (7) support systems
      (8) perceived quality of life
      (9) perceived regrets and guilt
     (10) spiritual distress
     (11) cultural diversity concerns that would affect patient's plan of care

L. Treatment history including
      (1) primary and secondary diagnoses
      (2) complications
      (3) hospitalizations
      (4) operative procedures
      (5) duration and types of replacement therapy and patient response to therapy
      (6) current medications and allergy history

Provide opportunities for patient to communicate feelings and concerns

Intervention

1. Assure completion of an evaluation by the interdisciplinary health care team
2. Encourage the patient and family to complete advance care planning and directives while offering additional resources for social, emotional, and spiritual support
3. Provide opportunities for patient to communicate feelings and concerns
4. Make appropriate referrals
5. Respectfully and carefully present palliative and end-of-life care goals for the patient and family to facilitate a dignified death that reflects the patient's wishes

Patient Teaching

Before teaching begins, consider health literacy and individualize the approach by considering patient's cultural and health beliefs, preferences, and wishes

1. Define palliative care. Explain that palliative care and hospice care do *not* mean that the patient must withdraw from dialysis. Each patient situation must be addressed individually
2. Reinforce that withdrawal from dialysis is the choice of the patient in consultation with his/her family and health care team and that it is not an abnormal occurrence
3. Explain the benefit of advance care planning and directives with the assurance that they can be changed by the patient at any time
4. Offer information and respond to questions regarding expectations, treatment goals, and dying trajectory
5. Provide appropriate resources and referrals as necessary

References

Centers for Medicare Services. (2009). *Conditions for coverage for dialysis.* Subpart C 494.70(a)(6) Standard: Patient Rights.

Chambers, E., Germain, M., & Brown, E. (2004). *Supportive care for the renal patient.* New York: Oxford University Press.

Kidney End of Life Coalition – http://kidneyeol.org

Kinzbrunner, B., Weinreb, N., & Policzer, J. (2002). *Twenty common problems: End of life care.* New York: McGraw-Hill.

Kuebler, K., & Berry, P. (2002). *End of life care: Clinical practice guidelines.* Philadelphia: Saunders.

Molzahn, A. (Ed.). (2006). *Contemporary nephrology nursing* (2nd ed., pp. 359-368). Pitman, NJ: American Nephrology Nurses' Association.

Renal Physicians Association (2010). *Clinical practice guideline on shared decision making in the appropriate initiation of and withdrawal from dialysis* (2nd ed.). Rockville, MD: Author.

World Health Organization. (1998). *WHO definition of palliative care.* Retrieved from http://www.who.int/cancer/palliative/definition/en

The following educational programs are available at www.prolibraries.com/anna

• ANNA End of Life Module 1 : Techniques to Facilitate Discussion for Advanced Care Planning

• ANNA End of Life Module 2: Ethical and Legal Aspects of Advanced Care Planning (ACP)

• ANNA End of Life Module 3: Cultural Diversity: Different Cultures, Different Solutions

• ANNA End of Life Module 4: Coordination of Hospice and Palliative Care in ESRD

• Toolkit for Nurturing Excellence at End-of-Life Transition (TNEEL) CD-rom. Funded by the Robert Wood Johnson Foundation; 1999-2003. Download at http://www.tneel.uic.edu/tneel.asp

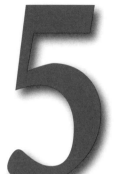

How to Use Nephrology Nursing Process of Care

The nephrology nursing process of care statements within this document are not intended to define a guideline for care and should not be construed as one. Neither should they be interpreted as prescribing an exclusive course of management. If a nephrology nurse is looking for prescriptive information regarding the management of the patient with kidney disease, the nurse should examine scholarly literature with the most current evidence-based information. Each nurse is responsible for evaluating appropriateness for the particular clinical situation.

The process of care section can be used to develop clinical skills checklists, performance evaluations, job descriptions, and professional development plans similar to the documents found in section 3.

The following forms are examples and should be modified to meet individual needs of the facility. Please go to **www.annanurse.org/StandardsForms** to download these documents for personal use. The documents are password protected. Enter the password **NephrologyNurse** when prompted.

Disclaimer

These forms were created for educational purposes only. They are intended to provide examples of the types of forms that administrators and nephrology registered nurses may want to use to incorporate the *Nephrology Nursing Scope and Standards of Practice* into clinical practice. The information provided is not intended to establish or replace forms provided by dialysis providers to their facilities. Please check with your dialysis facility management before implementing any form provided here.

It is the responsibility of the user to verify that the use of any of the forms does not violate any copyright laws.

Teaching Plan

At the QAPI meeting for the No Name Dialysis Center, the interdisciplinary team discussed the increase in the number of inadequate dialysis treatments. The nurse educator was tasked with developing a lesson plan for the direct patient care staff to specifically address inadequate dialysis. The nurse educator reviewed *Section 4: Nephrology Nursing Process of Care* in the *Nephrology Nursing Scope and Standards of Practice*, specifically *Standard 5b. Health Teaching and Health Promotion, Standard 8. Education,* and *Hemodialysis Adequacy.* The nurse educator also referenced the *Core Curriculum for Nephrology Nursing,* developed a lesson plan based on Bloom's taxonomy learning principles, and presented the plan to the interdisciplinary team for approval.

Teaching Plan

Date _____

Goal: To decrease the number of patients receiving inadequate dialysis treatments.

Lesson description:
Adequacy of the treatment impacts the patient on both a physical and psychological level. Both the registered nurse and the PCT have a role in delivering an "adequate" treatment to the patient. Patients present for treatment with different barriers impacting on the ability of the team to provide an adequate dialysis treatment. This lesson will discuss only the hemodialysis patient.

Learning principles:
• Students are likely to be motivated to learn things that are meaningful to them.
• Students are more likely to learn if they take active part in the practice geared to reach the objective.

Audience:
Direct patient care staff – includes both licensed and unlicensed staff.

Objectives	Teaching Strategies/ Level of Learning	Resources	Evaluation
At the end of this section, the learner will: • Explain what Kt/V and URR mean. *Cognitive – Comprehension – low to mid level* • State minimum goal for Kt/V and URR. *Cognitive – Knowledge – low level* • Identify at least three prescription changes that might be made to improve adequacy. *Cognitive – Knowledge – low level* • State the rationale for measuring adequacy of dialysis. *Cognitive – Knowledge – low level* • Verbalize the policy and procedure for adequacy blood draws on AV fistula patients. *Affective domain – Responding – low level* • Discuss possible solutions to complications of inadequate dialysis treatment. *Cognitive domain – Comprehension – low level*	**Lecture** – Direct teaching strategy used to give a foundation before discussing case studies. *Cognitive domain – Knowledge – low level; Comprehension – low level* **Questioning** – Questioning during the lecture increases interest and motivation. This will be an effective strategy for the mixed audience of licensed and unlicensed staff. Questions can differentiate the RN and PCT response to a specific patient situation. *Affective domain – Responding – low level* **Case studies** – Direct teaching strategy. The class will be divided into two groups to discuss the case studies and present findings to the entire class. *Cognitive domain – Application – medium to high level*	• PowerPoint presentation with LCD • Case studies and key	• Case study discussion • Quiz

Performance Criteria

The head hurse of the No Name Dialysis Center was asked by the director of nursing to develop performance criteria for CRRT. The head nurse reviewed the assessment and interventions indicated in the nephrology nursing process of care on CRRT from the *Nephrology Nursing Scope and Standards of Practice*. She developed a draft of the tool and presented it to the dialysis staff for input. They liked the tool and suggested an additional tool be developed using the items listed under the *Teaching for the Critical Care* nurse section.

No Name Dialysis Center				
Performance Criteria Checklist				
CONTINUOUS RENAL REPLACEMENT THERAPY (CRRT)				

Position:_____Department:_____

Employee's Name:_____Employee's Signature:_____

CRRT Criteria	Met / Not Met	Date & Evaluator		COMMENTS
		Date	Evaluator	
1. Checks for appropriate orders and consent before initiating treatment.	Y N			
2. Assesses vascular access site.	Y N			
3. Assesses patient's vital signs before initiating treatment.	Y N			
4. Attains pretreatment samples for lab test.	Y N			
5. If using blood pump; checks and sets:	Y N			
a. blood flow	Y N			
b. pressure monitor limits	Y N			
c. air detector	Y N			
6. Initiates treatment according to procedure.	Y N			
7. Administers anticoagulant or initiates infusion.	Y N			
a. Adjusts anticoagulation therapy based on patient's response and physician orders.	Y N			
b. Performs interventions specific to type of anticoagulant.	Y N			
8. Monitors the following during therapy:				
a. Blood pressure, pulse, temperature	Y N			
b. Cardiac rhythm, rate, dysrhythmias	Y N			
c. Level of consciousness, mentation	Y N			
d. Intravascular and extravascular volume status	Y N			
e. Respiratory status and oxygenation	Y N			
9. Responds appropriately to complications of treatment:				
a. Infection	Y N			
b. Hypoglycemia	Y N			
c. Hypothermia	Y N			
d. Blood leak	Y N			

AKI Scenario

The education department at No Name Dialysis Center has implemented a lab simulation program for critical care nurses. They contacted the dialysis department to develop a scenario for acute kidney injury (AKI). The dialysis nurse educator submitted a simulation scenario to ascertain the critical care nurses' knowledge of kidney replacement therapies. This is one example of several scenarios developed from identification of need to the completion of a CRRT treatment.

No Name Dialysis Center

AKI Simulation Scenario

Stage 3	Patient: *Norman Nephron*

Vital Signs & Comments	Participants should:	Debriefing Questions & Answers

BP: 100/60
HR: 124
RR: 32
SaO$_2$: 88
Temp: 39
Lungs: rales
Heart:
Rhythm: sinus tachycardia with occasional PVC
PAP:
CVP: 4
Wedge:
Notes: Patient complains of nausea, dizzy and weak, can't catch breath. Complains of severe pain in legs.
Pain scale a 6 out of 10
Wife still in home asking a lot of questions.
 	
If student asks, repeat K is 5.0
	1. Monitor fluid and electrolytes.
	2. Assess for infection.
	3. Administer medications as ordered.
	4. Contact dialysis nurse.
	5. Prepare patient for IJ catheter placement.
	6. Patient and/or family to sign consents.
	7. Explain procedure to patient and family.
		What are the treatments for AKI?
		   Diuretics – Loop, thiazides, potassium sparing, osmotic kidney replacement therapy
		What type of diuretic would the student anticipate the physician to order?
		   Loop diuretic – Lasix (furosemide) or Bumex (bumetanide)
		What are the different types of kidney replacement therapy?
		   Intermittent hemodialysis (IHD)
		   Continuous renal replacement therapy (CRRT)
		   Peritoneal dialysis (PD)
		   Kidney transplant
		What is the kidney replacement of choice for critically ill patient?
		   CRRT
		What is best choice for CRRT vascular access?
		   Internal jugular. Subclavian placement may cause stenosis and cause problems if vascular access needs to be placed for hemodialysis

Recommended Doctor's Orders	Lab Results	
1. Chest x-ray to verify placement of IJ catheter 2. Contact dialysis nurse for initiation of CRRT procedure	Hemoglobin (Hb)	8.9
	Hematocrit (Hct)	26.7
	PT	
	PTT	
	Sodium	
	Potassium	5.0
	Magnesium	
	Glucose	

Other Results	
X-ray:	Correct placement of IJ
CT-Scan:	
EKG:	

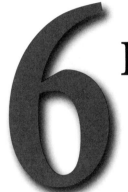

References

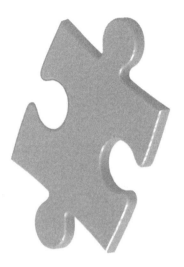

American Academy of Sleep Medicine – www.aasmnet.org

American Association of Critical-Care Nurses Certification Corporation. (2003). *Synergy model – Background*. Retrieved from http://www.aacn.org/wd/certifications/content/synmodel.pcms?pid= 1&&menu=Certification#Basic

American Diabetes Association. (2004a). Diagnosis and classification of diabetes mellitus. *Diabetes Care, 27*(Suppl. 1), S5-S10.

American Diabetes Association. (2004b). Nephropathy in diabetes. *Diabetes Care, 27*(Suppl. 1), S79-S83.

American Diabetes Association. (2004c). Nutrition principles and recommendations in diabetes. *Diabetes Care, 27*(Suppl. 1), S36-S46.

American Diabetes Association. (2010). Diagnosis and classification of diabetes mellitus. *Diabetes Care, 33(S62-69).* doi: 10.2337/dcro-S062.

American Nurses Association. (2008). Professional role competence position statement. Retrieved from http://nursingworld.org/MainMenuCategories/HealthcareandPolicyIssues/ ANAPositionStatements/practice/PositionStatementProfessionalRoleCompetence.aspx

American Nurses Association. (2010a). *Guide to the code of ethics for nurses: Interpretation and application.* Washington, DC: Nursesbooks.org

American Nurses Association. (2010b). *Nursing: Scope and standards of practice* (2nd ed). Silver Spring, MD: Nursesbooks.org.

American Nurses Association. (2010c). *Nursing's social policy statement: The essence of the profession.* Silver Spring, MD: Nursesbooks.org.

American Nephrology Nurses' Association. (2002). *Advanced practice nurse standards of professional performance.* Pitman, NJ: Author.

American Nephrology Nurses' Association. (2004a). *ANNA fact sheet.* Pitman, NJ: Author.

American Nephrology Nurses' Association. (2004b). *Discover nephrology nursing.* Pitman, NJ: Author.

American Nephrology Nurses' Association. (2004c). *Minimum preparation for entry into nursing practice.* Pitman, NJ: Author.

American Society for Apheresis. (2010, April 14). *American Society for Apheresis guidelines. Resources for apheresis professionals.* Retrieved from http://www.apheresis.org/asfa_guidelines

APRN Joint Dialogue Group. (2008). *Consensus model for APRN regulation: Licensure, accreditation, certification and education.* Retrieved from http://www.nursingworld.org/ConsensusModelforAPRN

Association for the Advancement of Medical Instrumentation – www.aami.org/standards

Blake, P.G., & Diaz-Buxo, J. (2001). Adequacy of peritoneal dialysis and chronic peritoneal dialysis prescription. In J.T. Daugirdas, P.G. Blake, & T.S. Ing. (Eds.), *Handbook of dialysis* (3rd ed., pp. 343-360). Philadelphia: Lippincott Williams & Wilkins.

Board of Higher Education & Massachusetts Organization of Nurse Executives. (2006). *Creativity and connections: Building the framework for the Future of Nursing Education.* Report from the Invitational Working Session, March 23–24, 2006. Burlington, MA: Massachusetts Organization of Nurse Executives. Retrieved from http://www.mass.edu/currentinit/documents/ NursingCreativityAndConnections.pdf

Campaign to Prevent Antimicrobial Resistance in Dialysis Patients. Centers for Disease Control and Prevention. http://www.cdc.gov/drugresistance/healthcare/patients.htm#dialysis

Coleman, B., & Merrill, J.P. (1952). The artificial kidney. *American Journal of Nursing, 52*(3), 327-329.

Centers for Disease Control and Prevention. (1995). Recommendations for preventing the spread of vancomycin resistance recommendations of the Hospital Infection Control Practices Advisory Committee (HICPAC). *Morbidity and Mortality Weekly Report, 44*(RR12).

Centers for Disease Control and Prevention. (2001). Recommendations for preventing transmission of infections among chronic hemodialysis patients. *Morbidity and Mortality Weekly Report, 50*(RR-5).

Centers for Disease Control and Prevention. (2002). Guidelines for the prevention of intravascular catheter-related infections. *Morbidity and Mortality Weekly Report, Recommendations and Reports, 51*(RR-10A), 1-29.

Centers for Disease Control and Prevention. (2003). Guidelines for laboratory testing and result reporting of antibody to hepatitis C. *Morbidity and Mortality Weekly Report, 52*(RR03), 1-16.

Centers for Disease Control and Prevention. (2005a). Guidelines for preventing the transmission of *Mycobacterium tuberculosis* in health-care settings. *Morbidity and Mortality Weekly Report, 54*(RR-17).

Centers for Disease Control and Prevention. (2005b). Guidelines for the investigation of contacts of persons with infectious tuberculosis: Recommendations from the National Tuberculosis Controllers Association and the CDC. *Morbidity and Mortality Weekly Report, 54*(RR-15).

Centers for Disease Control and Prevention. (2010). Updated guidelines for using interferon gamma release assays to detect *Mycobacterium tuberculosis* infection. *Morbidity and Mortality Weekly Report, 59(RR-5).*

Centers for Medicare and Medicaid Services. (2008). *Conditions for coverage for end stage renal disease facilities: Final rule, Federal Register.* Retrieved from http://www.cms.gov/cfcsandcops/downloads/esrdfinalrule0415.pdf

Centers for Medicare Services and Medicaid Services. (2009). *Conditions for coverage for dialysis.* Subpart C 494.70(a)(6) Standard: Patient Rights.

Chambers, E., Germain, M., & Brown, E. (2004). *Supportive care for the renal patient.* New York: Oxford University Press.

Chobanian, A.V., Bakris, G.L., Black, H.R., Cushman, W.C., Green, L.A., Izzo, J.L., Jr., Jones, D.W., Materson, B.J., Oparil, S., Wright, J.T., Jr., & Rocella, E.J. National Heart, Lung, and Blood Institute Joint National Committee on Prevention, Detection, Evaluation, and Treatment of High Blood Pressure. (2004). The seventh report of the Joint National Committee on Prevention, Detection, Evaluation, and Treatment of High Blood Pressure: The JNC 7 report. *Journal of the American Medical Association, 289*(19), 2560-2572.

Counts, C. (Ed.). (2008). *Core curriculum for nephrology nursing* (5th ed.). Pitman, NJ: American Nephrology Nurses' Association.

Dinwiddie, L.C. (2008). Vascular access for hemodialysis. In C. Counts (Ed.), *Core curriculum for nephrology nursing* (5th ed., pp. 735-764). Pitman, NJ: American Nephrology Nurses' Association.

Expert Panel on Detection, Evaluation and Treatment of High Blood Cholesterol in Adults (ATP III Guidelines). (2003). Executive summary of the third report of the national cholesterol education program (NCEP) expert panel on detection, evaluation, and treatment of high blood cholesterol in adults (Adult Treatment Panel III). *Journal of the American Medical Association, 285*, 2486-2497.

Finkelstein, F., & Finkelstein, S. (2000). Depression in chronic dialysis patients: Assessment and treatment. *Nephrology Dialysis Transplantation, 15*(12), 1911-1913.

Fulton, B.J., & Cameron, E.M. (1989). Perspectives on our beginnings: 1962-1979. *ANNA Journal, 16*(3), 201-203.

Georgetown University. Bright futures. Retrieved from www.brightfutures.org/healthcheck/resources/maturity.htm

Gokal, R., Alexander, S., Ash, S., Chen, T.W., Danielson, A., Holmes, C., Joffe, P., Moncrief, J., Nichols, K., Piraino, B., Prowant, B., Slingeneyer, A., Stegmayr, B., Twardowski, Z., & Vas, S. (1998). Peritoneal catheters and exit-site practices toward optimum peritoneal access: 1998 update. *Peritoneal Dialysis International, 18*(1), 11-33.

Hays, R.D., Kallich, J.D., Mapes, D.L., Coons, S.J., Amin, N., Carter, W.B., & Kamberg, C. (1997). *Kidney disease quality of life short form (KDQOL-SF), Version 1.3: A manual for use and scoring,* P-7994. Santa Monica, CA: RAND.

Hoffart, N. (1989). Nephrology nursing 1915-1970: A historical study of the integration of technology and care. *ANNA Journal, 16*(3), 169-178.

Hudson, S., & Prowant, B. (2005). *Nephrology nursing standards of practice and guidelines for care.* Pitman, NJ: American Nephrology Nurses' Association.

Kam-Tao, P., Szeto, C.C., Piraino, B., Bernardini, J., Figueiredo, A.E., Gupta, A., Johnson, D.W., Kuijper, E.J., Lye, W.C., Salzer, W, Schafer, F., & Struijk, D.G. (2010). Peritoneal dialysis-related infections recommendations: 2010 update. *Peritoneal Dialysis International, 30*, 393-423.

Kauffman, J., Myers, L., Rohe, R., & Axley, B. (2009). Clinical application: CQI aspects of the Therapeutic Apheresis Program. In B. Axley & K. Robbins (Eds.), *Applying continuous quality improvement in clinical practice* (2nd ed., pp. 125-130). Pitman, NJ: American Nephrology Nurses' Association.

Kidney Disease: Improving Global Outcomes. (2009). Clinical practice guidelines for the diagnosis, evaluation, prevention, and treatment of chronic kidney disease-mineral and bone disorder (CKD-MBD). *Kidney International, 76*(Suppl. 113); S 1-130.

Keane, W.F., Bailie, G.R., Boeschoten, E., Gokal, R., Golper, T.A., Holmes, C.J., Kawaguchi, Y., Piraino, B., Riella, M., & Vas, S. (2000). Adult peritoneal dialysis-related peritonitis treatment recommendations: 2000 Update. *Peritoneal Dialysis International, 20*(6), 828-829.

Kidney End of Life Coalition – http://kidneyeol.org

Kidney Disease Quality of Life Working Group – www.gim.med.ucla.edu/kdqol

Kinzbrunner, B., Weinreb, N., & Policzer, J. (2002). *Twenty common problems: End of life care.* New York: McGraw-Hill.

Korbet, S. M., & Kronfol, N.O. (2001). Acute peritoneal dialysis prescription. In J.T. Daugirdas, P.G. Blake, & T.S. Ing. (Eds.), *Handbook of dialysis* (3rd ed., pp. 333-342). Philadelphia: Lippincott Williams & Wilkins.

Kuebler, K., Berry, P., & Heidrich, D. (2002). *End of life care: Clinical practice guidelines.* Philadelphia: Saunders.

McKenna, R. (Coordinator). (2001). *Guidelines for education, training and competency in apheresis.* Sydney: Australian and New Zealand Apheresis Association. Retrieved from http://www.anzsbt .org.au/publications/documents/ANZAA_Apheresis_Education_Guidelines_Jun01.pdf

Mitchell, S. (2002). Estimated dry weight (EDW): Aiming for accuracy. *Nephrology Nursing Journal, 29*(5), 421-428.

Molzahn, A. (Ed.). (2006). *Contemporary nephrology nursing* (2nd ed., pp. 359-368). Pitman, NJ: American Nephrology Nurses' Association.

National Kidney Foundation. (2000a). K/DOQI clinical practice guidelines for anemia of chronic kidney disease: Update 2000. *American Journal of Kidney Diseases, 37*(1)(Suppl. 1), S182-S238.

National Kidney Foundation. (2000b). K/DOQI clinical practice guidelines for nutrition in chronic renal failure. *American Journal of Kidney Diseases, 35*(6)(Suppl. 2), S1-S140. Erratum in: (2001). *American Journal of Kidney Diseases, 38*(4), 917.

National Kidney Foundation. (2001). K/DOQI clinical practice guidelines for peritoneal dialysis adequacy. *American Journal of Kidney Diseases, 37*(1)(Suppl. 1), S65-S136.

National Kidney Foundation. (2002). K/DOQI clinical practice guidelines for chronic kidney disease: Evaluation, classification and stratification. *American Journal of Kidney Diseases, 39*(2)(Suppl. 1), S1-S266.

National Kidney Foundation. (2003a). KDOQI clinical practice guidelines for bone metabolism and disease in chronic kidney disease. *American Journal of Kidney Diseases, 42*(4)(Suppl. 3), S1-S201.

National Kidney Foundation. (2003b). NKF-KDOQI clinical practice guidelines for managing dyslipidemias in chronic kidney disease. *American Journal of Kidney Diseases, 41*(4)(Suppl. 3), S1-S91.

National Kidney Foundation. (2004). K/DOQI clinical practice guidelines on hypertension and antihypertensive agents in chronic kidney disease. *American Journal of Kidney Diseases, 43*(5)(Suppl. 1), S1-S290.

National Kidney Foundation. (2006a). KDOQI clinical practice guidelines and clinical practice recommendations for anemia of chronic kidney disease. *American Journal of Kidney Diseases, 47*(5)(Suppl. 3), S1-S145.

National Kidney Foundation. (2006b). NKF-KDOQI clinical practice guidelines for blood pressure management and use of antihypertensive agents in chronic kidney disease. *American Journal of Kidney Diseases, 48*(1)(Suppl. 1), S1-183.

National Kidney Foundation. (2006c). NKF-KDOQI clinical practice guidelines for hemodialysis adequacy. *American Journal of Kidney Diseases, 48*(1)(Suppl. 1), S13-97.

National Kidney Foundation. (2006d). NKF-KDOQI clinical practice guidelines for vascular access: Update 2006. *American Journal of Kidney Diseases, 48*(1)(Suppl. 1), S176-S307.

National Kidney Foundation. (2007a). KDOQI clinical practice guidelines for anemia of chronic kidney disease: 2007 update of hemoglobin target. *American Journal of Kidney Diseases, 50*(3), 471-530.

National Kidney Foundation. (2007b). *Kidney Disease Outcomes Quality Initiative.* Retrieved from http://www.kidney.org/professionals/kdoqi/guidelines_commentaries.cfm

National Sleep Foundation – www.sleepfoundation.org

Nephrology Nursing Certification Commission. (2005). Pitman, NJ. Retrieved from http://www.nncc-exam.org

Newhouse, R.P. (2010). Clinical guidelines for nursing practice: Are we there yet? *Journal of Nursing Administration, 40*(2), 57-59.

Nielsen, S., Knepper, M.A., Kwon, T.H., & Frokiaer, J. (2004). Regulation of water balance. In B.M. Brenner (Ed.), *Brenner and Rector's the kidney* (7th ed., Vol. 1), 109-134. Philadelphia: Saunders.

Oreopoulos, D.G., & Rao, P. (2001). Assessing peritoneal ultrafiltration, solute transport, and volume status. In J.T. Daugirdas, P.G. Blake, & T.S. Ing. (Eds.), *Handbook of dialysis* (3rd ed., pp. 361-372). Philadelphia: Lippincott Williams & Wilkins.

Parker, J. (1998). Nephrology nursing as a specialty. In J. Parker (Ed.), *Contemporary nephrology nursing* (pp. 3-23). Pitman, NJ: American Nephrology Nurses' Association.

Parker, K.P., Kutner, N.G., Bliwise, D., Bailey, J.L., & Rye, D.B. (2003). Nocturnal sleep, daytime sleepiness, and quality of life in stable patients on hemodialysis. *Health and Quality of Life Outcomes, 1*, 68. doi: 10.1186/1477-7525-1-68. Retrieved from http://www.ncbi.nlm.nih.gov/pmc/articles/PMC320494

Passow, J., Pineda, A., & Burgstaler, E. (1984). Responsibilities of the registered nurse in the apheresis laboratory. Journal of Clinical Apheresis. Retrieved from http://www3.interscience.wiley.com/journal/113466992/abstract

Pender, N.J., Murdaugh, C.L., & Parsons, M.A. (2005). *Health promotion in nursing practice* (5th ed.). Upper Saddle River, NJ: Prentice Hall.

Performance, excellence, and accountability in kidney care – www.kidneycarequality.com

Renal Physicians Association (2010). *Clinical practice guideline on shared decision making in the appropriate initiation of and withdrawal from dialysis* (2nd ed.). Rockville, MD: Author.

Rosenthal, K. (2010). *Introduction to apheresis.* Retrieved from http://www.resourcenurse.com/about.html

Siegel, J., Rhinehart, E., Jackson, M., Chiarello, L., & the Healthcare Infection Control Practices Advisory Committee, Centers for Disease Control and Prevention. (2007). *Guideline for isolation precautions: Preventing transmission of infectious agents in healthcare settings.* Retrieved from http://www.cdc.gov/hicpac/2007IP/2007isolationPrecautions.html

Simmons, L. (2009). Dorothea Orem's self care theory as related to nursing practice in hemodialysis. *Nephrology Nursing Journal, 36*(4), 419-421.

Smith, K.S. (1994). ANNA's involvement in legislative arena targets all levels of government. In *ANNA: 1969-1994. Celebrating 25 years of service to the nephrology community* (p. 20). Pitman, NJ: American Nephrology Nurses' Association.

Styles, M.M., Schumann, M.J.Bickford, C.J., & White, K. (2008). Specialization and credentialing in nursing revisited: Understanding the issues, advancing the profession. Silver Spring, MD: Nursesbooks.org.

Tanner, J.M. (1962). *Growth at adolescence* (2nd ed.). Oxford, England: Blackwell Scientific Publications.

Thomas-Hawkins, C., Denno, M., Currier, H., & Wick, G. (2003). Staff nurses perceptions of the work environment in free standing hemodialysis facilities. *Nephrology Nursing Journal, 30*(24), 377-386.

Thomas-Hawkins, C., Flynn, L., & Clarke, S. (2008). Relationships between registered nurse staffing, process of nursing care, and nurse-reported patient outcomes in chronic hemodialysis units. *Nephrology Nursing Journal, 35*(2), 123-131.

Twardowski, Z.J., & Prowant, B.F. (1996). Appearance and classification of healing peritoneal catheter exit sites. *Peritoneal Dialysis International, 16*(Suppl. 3), S71-S93.

Uhlig, K., Berns, J., Kestenbaum, B., Kumar, R., Leonard, M., Martin, K., Sprague, S., & Goldfarb, S. (2009). US commentary on the 2009 KDIGO clinical practice guideline for diagnosis, evaluation, and treatment of CKD-mineral and bone disorder (CKD-MBD). *American Journal of Kidney Disease, 55*(5), 773-799.

Ulrich, B.T. (2006). Professional nephrology nursing: The specialty, the community, and the nursing roles. In A. Molzahn (Ed.), *Contemporary nephrology nursing* (2nd ed.). Pitman, NJ: American Nephrology Nurses' Association.

United States Renal Data System. (2009). *USRDS annual data report.* Retrieved from http://www.usrds.org

VanBuskirk, S. (2003). Nephrology nursing shortage and solutions invitational summit: Task forces to follow up on defined projects. *Nephrology Nursing Journal, 30*(4), 410.

Warady, B.A., Schaefer, F., Holloway, M., Alexander, S., Kandert, M., Piraino, B., Salusky, I., Tranaeus, A., Divino, J., Honda, M., Mujais, S., & Verrina, E. International Society for Peritoneal Dialysis (ISPD) Advisory Committee on Peritonitis Management in Pediatric Patients. (2000). Consensus guidelines for the treatment of peritonitis in pediatric patients receiving peritoneal dialysis. *Peritoneal Dialysis International, 20*(6), 610-624. Erratum in (2001). *Peritoneal Dialysis International, 21*(1), 6.

World Health Organization. (1998). *WHO definition of palliative care.* Retrieved from http://www.who.int/cancer/palliative/definition/en/

Wiggins, J. (2009). Integrated care of the elderly with ESKD. Geriatric Nephrology Curriculum. American Society of Nephrology. Retrieved from www.asn-online.org

Williams, H.F., Waack, T., & Axley, B. (2009). Clinical application: CQI in continuous renal replacement therapy. In B. Axley & K.C. Robbins (Eds.), *Applying continuous quality improvement in clinical practice* (2nd ed., pp. 133-139). Pitman, NJ: American Nephrology Nurses' Association.

Wilson, B., Spittal, J., Heidenheim, P., Herman, M., Leonard, M., Johnston, A., Lindsay, R., & Moist, L. (2006). Screening for depression in chronic hemodialysis patients: Comparison of the Beck Depression Inventory, primary nurse, and nephrology team. *Hemodialysis International, 10*(1), 35-41.

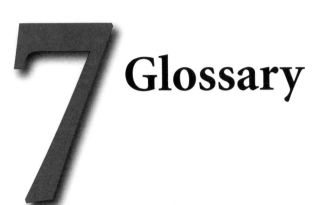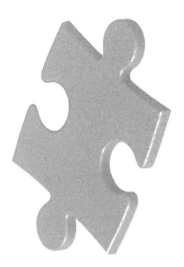

Glossary

AAMI

The Association of the Advancement of Medical Instrumentation. This organization sets the standards and recommended practice for dialysis machines, reuse of dialyzers, electrical safety, monitoring and culturing of machines and water systems, cleaning of machines, quality of water used for dialysis and methodology for bacterial sampling.

Advanced practice registered nurses (APRN)

A nurse who has completed an accredited graduate-level education program preparing her or him for the role of certified nurse practitioner, certified registered nurse anesthetist, certified nurse-midwife, or clinical nurse specialist; has passed a national certification examination that measures the APRN role and population-focused competencies; maintains continued competence as evidenced by recertification; and is licensed to practice as an APRN. (Adapted from APRN JDG, 2008.)

Assessment

A systematic, dynamic process by which the registered nurse, through interaction with the patient, family, groups, communities, populations, and healthcare providers, collects and analyzes data. Assessment may include the following dimensions: physical, psychological, sociocultural, spiritual, cognitive, functional abilities, developmental, economic, and lifestyle.

Autonomy

The capacity of a nurse to determine her or his own actions through independent choice, including demonstration of competence, within the full scope of nursing practice.

Caregiver

A person who provides direct care for another, such as a child, dependent adult, the disabled, or the chronically ill.

Chronic kidney disease (CKD)

A progressive loss in kidney function over a period of months or years. It is divided into stages based on glomerular filtration rate.

Code of ethics (nursing)

A list of provisions that makes explicit the primary goals, values, and obligations of the nursing profession and expresses its values, duties, and commitments to the society of which it is a part. In the United States, nurses abide by and adhere to the *Guide to the Code of Ethics for Nurses: Interpretation and Application* (ANA, 2010).

Collaboration

A professional health care partnership grounded in a reciprocal and respectful recognition and acceptance of: each partner's unique expertise, power, and sphere of influence and responsibilities; the commonality of goals; the mutual safeguarding of the legitimate interest of each party; and, the advantages of such a relationship.

Competency

An expected and measureable level of nursing performance that integrates knowledge, skills, abilities, and judgment, based on established scientific knowledge and expectations for nursing practice.

Continuity of care

An interdisciplinary process that includes healthcare consumers, families, and other stakeholders in the development of a coordinated plan of care. This process facilitates the patient's transition between settings and health care providers, based on changing needs and available resources.

Delegation

The transfer of responsibility for the performance of a task from one individual to another while retaining accountability for the outcome. Example: the RN, in delegating a task to an assistive individual, transfers the responsibility for the performance of the task but retains professional accountability for the overall care.

Diagnosis

A clinical judgment about the healthcare consumer's response to actual or potential health conditions or needs. The diagnosis provides the basis for determination of a plan to achieve expected outcomes. Registered nurses use nursing and medical diagnoses depending upon educational and clinical preparation and legal authority.

Environment

The surrounding context, milieu, conditions, or atmosphere in which a registered nurse practices.

Environmental health

Aspects of human health, including quality of life, that are determined by physical, chemical, biological, social, and psychological problems in the environment. It also refers to the theory and practice of assessing, correcting, controlling, and preventing those factors in the environment that can potentially affect adversely the health of present and future generations.

ESRD Networks

The End-Stage Renal Disease Networks were established in 1978 to oversee dialysis centers to ensure patients receive quality care. They collect data, implement quality improvement programs, establish grievance procedures, and provide resources.

Evaluation

The process of determining the progress toward attainment of expected outcomes, including the effectiveness of care.

Expected outcomes

End results that are measurable, desirable, and observable, and translate into observable behaviors.

Evidence-based practice

A scholarly and systematic problem-solving paradigm that results in the delivery of high quality health care.

Family

Family of origin or significant others as identified by the healthcare consumer.

Health

An experience that is often expressed in terms of wellness and illness, and may occur in the presence or absence of disease or injury.

Healthcare consumer

The person, client, family, group, community, or population that is the focus of attention and to whom the registered nurse is providing services as sanctioned by the state regulatory bodies.

Health care providers

Individuals with special expertise who provide health care services or assistance to patients. They may include nurses, physicians, psychologists, social workers, nutritionist/dietitians, and various therapists.

Illness

The subjective experience of discomfort.

Implementation

Activities such as teaching, monitoring, providing, counseling, delegating, and coordinating.

Information

Data that is interpreted, organized, or structured.

Interdisciplinary

Reliant on the overlapping knowledge, skills, and abilities of each professional team member. Consists of, at a minimum, the patient or the patient's designee (if the patient chooses), a registered nurse, a physician treating the patient for ESRD (APRN or PA may substitute for physician), a social worker, and a dietitian.

K/DOQI

National Kidney Foundation's Guidelines, Kidney Disease Outcomes Quality Initiative

KRT

Kidney replacement therapies; new term being used in place of renal replacement therapies (RRT). These terms identify all therapies used to treat kidney disease, which include dialysis, transplantation, and palliative care.

Medical home

Care that uses primary care providers to ensure the delivery of coordinated, comprehensive care.

Medicare ESRD Program

The Medicare ESRD Program was established in 1972. The program provides benefits to patients with kidney disease who are entitled to Social Security benefits.

Nephrology nursing

Nephrology nursing is a specialty practice addressing the protection, promotion, and optimization of health and well-being of individuals with kidney disease. This is achieved through the prevention and treatment of illness and injury, and the alleviation of suffering through patient, family, and community advocacy.

Nursing

The protection, promotion, and optimization of health and abilities; prevention of illness and injury; alleviation of suffering through the diagnosis and treatment of human response; and advocacy in the care of individuals, families, communities, and populations.

Nursing practice

The collective professional activities of nurses that is characterized by the interrelations of human responses, theory application, nursing actions, and outcomes.

Nursing process

A critical thinking model used by nurses that is characterized by the integration of the singular, concurrent actions of these six components: assessment, diagnosis, identification of outcomes, planning, implementation, and evaluation.

Patient

See Healthcare consumer

Peer review

A collegial, systematic, and periodic process by which registered nurses are held accountable for practice and which fosters the refinement of one's knowledge, skills, and decision making at all levels and in all areas of practice.

Plan

A comprehensive outline of the components that need to be addressed to attain expected outcomes.

Quality

The degree to which health services for patients, families, groups, communities, or populations increase the likelihood of desired outcomes and are consistent with current professional knowledge.

Registered nurse (RN)

An individual registered or licensed by a state, commonwealth, territory, government, or other regulatory body to practice as a registered nurse.

Scope of nephrology nursing practice

The description of the who, what, where, when, why, and how of nephrology nursing practice. When considered in conjunction with the *Nephrology Nursing Standards of Professional Practice* and the *ANA Code of Ethics for Nurses*, comprehensively describes the competent level of nephrology nursing.

Scope of nursing practice

The description of the who, what, where, when, why, and how of nursing practice that addresses the range of nursing practice activities common to all registered nurses. When considered in conjunction with the Standards of Professional Nursing Practice and the Code of Ethics for Nurses, comprehensively describes the competent level of nursing common to all registered nurses.

Standards

Authoritative statements defined and promoted by the profession by which the quality of practice, service, or education can be evaluated.

Standards of nephrology practice

Describe a competent level of nephrology nursing care as demonstrated by the nursing process.

Standards of professional nursing practice

Authoritative statements of the duties that all registered nurses, regardless of role, population, or specialty, are expected to perform competently.

Standards of professional performance

Describe a competent level of behavior in the professional role.

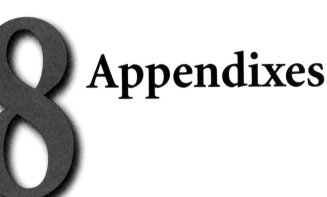

Appendixes

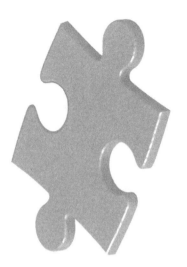

Position Statements

Appendix A   Delegation of Nursing Care Activities

Appendix B   Advanced Practice in Nephrology Nursing

Appendix C   Certification in Nephrology Nursing

Appendix D   ANNA Health Policy Statement

Publications

Appendix E   Principles and Elements of a Healthful Practice/
Work Environment

Appendix F   Reference Card from the Seventh Report of the Joint
National Committee on Prevention, Detection, Evaluation,
and Treatment of High Blood Pressure (JNC 7)

Appendix A Delegation of Nursing Care Activities (page 1 of 3)

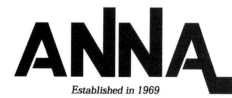

Position Statement

American Nephrology Nurses' Association

Established in 1969

Delegation of Nursing Care Activities

The American Nephrology Nurses' Association (ANNA) believes every patient has the right to professional nursing care that encompasses all aspects of the nursing process and meets or exceeds the *ANNA Nephrology Nursing Standards of Practice and Guidelines for Care* and Centers for Medicare and Medicaid Services (CMS) Conditions for Coverage and will comply with the regulation of the state in which they are employed. This is to include, but is not limited to, assessment of patient needs, the development of a plan of nursing care, implementation of nursing interventions, and the monitoring and evaluation of nursing actions. The ultimate goal of the nursing process is to effect positive patient outcomes. ANNA recognizes that achievement of favorable patient outcomes is a collaborative effort between all members of the interdisciplinary team.

It is the position of ANNA that:

- The registered nurse must never delegate a nursing care activity that requires:

  a. The knowledge and expertise derived from completion of a nursing education program and the specialized skill, judgment and decision-making of a registered nurse
  b. An understanding of the core nephrology nursing principles necessary to recognize and manage real or potential complications that may result in an adverse outcome to the health and safety of the patient.

- Delegation of nursing care activities to licensed practical/vocational nurses (LPN/LVNs) shall comply with the following criteria:

  a. The registered nurse must complete an assessment of the patient's nursing care needs prior to delegating any nursing intervention.
  b. The registered nurse shall be accountable and responsible for all delegated nursing care activities or interventions, and she/he must remain present in the patient care area for ongoing monitoring and evaluation of the patient's response to the therapy.
  c. The patient care activities must be within the scope of practice delineated by the Board of LPN/LVN for the state in which the nurses are practicing and must not require the LPN/LVN to exercise nursing judgment beyond the scope of that practice act.
  d. The registered nurse shall have either instructed the LPN/LVN in the delegated nursing care activity or verified the individual's competency to perform the activity. Clinical competency of these individual's will be documented and available, and verified at least annually.

ANNA National Office   East Holly Avenue, Box 56   Pitman, NJ 08071-0056
Phone: 888-600-ANNA (2662) or 856-256-2320 **Fax**: 856-589-7463 **Email**: anna@ajj.com **Website**: www.annanurse.org

Appendix A Delegation of Nursing Care Activities (page 2 of 3)

Page 2
Delegation of Nursing Care Activities

- Delegation of nursing care activities to unlicensed assistive personnel shall comply with the following criteria:

    a. The registered nurse must complete an assessment of the patient's nursing care needs prior to delegating any nursing care activities or interventions.
    b. The registered nurse shall be accountable and responsible for all delegated nursing care activities or interventions, and she/he must remain present in the patient care area for the ongoing monitoring and evaluation of the patient's response to the therapy.
    c. The registered nurse shall have either instructed the unlicensed assistive personnel in the delegated nursing care activity or verified the individual's competency to perform the activity. Clinical competency and knowledge of these individuals will be documented and available, and verified at least annually.
    d. Since unlicensed assistive personnel practicing in nephrology do not have a recognized scope of practice delineated by an approved state board of occupational regulations, the registered nurse shall be responsible for the ongoing evaluation of the performance of these individuals and supervision of all the nursing care activities performed by them.
    e. Administration of medication is a nursing responsibility requiring knowledge of the indications, pharmacokinetic action, potential adverse reactions, correct dosage and contraindications, and it is beyond the scope of practice of unlicensed assistive personnel. Administration of medications by unlicensed assistive personnel shall be limited to those medications considered part of the routine hemodialysis treatment, that is, normal saline and heparin via the extracorporeal circuit and intradermal lidocaine (as allowed by individual state practice act).
    f. Administration of any blood products and/or intravenous medications by infusion is a nursing responsibility and beyond the scope of practice of unlicensed assistive personnel.

- The registered nurse is legally accountable and clinically responsible for the complete documentation of the entire nursing process. As certain aspects of the nursing care activities or interventions may be delegated to other personnel, the registered nurse also retains the legal accountability and clinical responsibility for these activities.

Background and Rationale

The relationship between the registered nurse and the patient constitutes a legal and binding contract. (The existence of this contract has been established through case law.)

ANNA also recognizes potential contributions to the care of nephrology patients by LPN/LVN and unlicensed assistive personnel. The scope of practice of the registered nurse may allow the delegation of ONLY selected nursing care activities or interventions to these licensed and unlicensed assistive personnel.

References

American Nurses Association (ANA). (2005). *Principles of delegation.* Washington, DC: American Nurses Publishing.

American Nurses Association (ANA). (2003). *Nursing scope and standards of practice.* Washington, DC: American Nurses Publishing.

ANNA National Office   East Holly Avenue, Box 56   Pitman, NJ 08071-0056
Phone: 888-600-ANNA (2662) or 856-256-2320   **Fax**: 856-589-7463   **Email**: anna@ajj.com   **Website**: http://www.annanurse.org

Appendix A   Delegation of Nursing Care Activities (page 3 of 3)

Page 3
Delegation of Nursing Care Activities

American Nurses Association (ANA). (2003). *Nursing's social policy statement* (2nd ed.). Washington, DC: American Nurses Publishing.

American Nurses Association (ANA). (2001). *Code of ethics for nurses with interpretive statements.* Washington, DC: American Nurses Publishing.

Anthony, M.K., Standing, T., & Hertz, J.E. (2000). Factors influencing outcomes after delegation to unlicensed assistive personnel. *Journal of Nursing Administration, 30*(10), 474-481.

Centers for Medicare & Medicaid Services (CMS). (2008). Final rule displayed at: www.cms.hhs.gov/CFCsAndCoPs/downloads/ESRDdisplayfinalrule.pdf.

Adopted by the ANNA Board of Directors in February 1986
Revised and/or reaffirmed biennially from 1987-2010
Most recently revised: July 2010

ANNA Position Statements are reviewed and reaffirmed biennially.

Appendix B Advanced Practice in Nephrology Nursing (page 1 of 2)

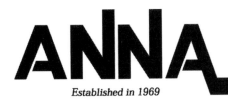

Position Statement

American Nephrology Nurses' Association

Established in 1969

Advanced Practice in Nephrology Nursing

The present healthcare environment mandates high quality, cost-effective, patient and family focused care. Trends in the incidence and prevalence of CKD indicate that this patient population will continue to grow. This growth will be accompanied by an increased need for qualified health care providers who have the knowledge and skills to manage, provide, and coordinate the care of this complex patient population. APNs in Nephrology Nursing are qualified providers to meet the needs of this patient population.

It is the position of ANNA that:

- The advanced practice nurse in nephrology, transplantation and related therapies, by virtue of education, training, and certification, as well as documented competencies, is able to provide safe, competent, high-quality care in a cost-effective manner. In addition, the advanced practice nurse focuses on promoting the health and well being of patients and on preventing disease and/or its subsequent complications along the entire continuum of kidney dysfunction. The advanced practice nurse may provide and coordinate the care of patients with kidney disease in both the acute and chronic care settings and across all treatment modalities. The advanced practice nephrology nurse is an integral member of the healthcare team and works collaboratively with other healthcare professionals to assure the highest standard of quality care.

- The American Nephrology Nurses' Association (ANNA) endorses the title "Advanced Practice Nurse" (APN) to designate both the clinical nurse specialist (CNS) and nurse practitioner (NP) roles. This is in agreement with the American Nurses Association (ANA), which recognizes four principal types of APNs, namely, clinical nurse specialist, nurse practitioner, certified nurse midwife, and certified registered nurse anesthetist. The requirement for the advanced practice nurse in nephrology nursing is a graduate degree in nursing, advanced content in the clinical specialty, and experience in nursing. Competencies of the advanced practice nurse in nephrology include the ability to:

a. provide expert nursing care to individuals with varying degrees of kidney impairment
b. assess the healthcare needs of individuals, families, groups and communities
c. use the nursing process to diagnose, plan, implement, and manage care as well as to evaluate the outcomes of that care
d. focus on care that promotes health, prevents kidney disease, presents and/or manages the complications of acute and chronic disease and prevents disability
e. assist patients and families with modality choices (including hemodialysis, PD, transplant, and conservative management)
f. support the palliative care and end-of-life needs of patients and their families
g. provide and coordinate care for complex patient, family, and community populations
h. manage acute and chronic kidney disease in a variety of healthcare settings
i. prescribe, administer, and evaluate pharmacologic and non-pharmacologic therapeutic treatment regimens
j. explore, test, and advance scientific theories upon which nursing practice is based
k. independently assess, conceptualize, and diagnose complex health problems

---

ANNA National Office   East Holly Avenue, Box 56   Pitman, NJ 08071-0056
Phone: 888-600-ANNA (2662) or 856-256-2320   **Fax**: 856-589-7463   **Email**: anna@ajj.com   **Website**: http://www.annanurse.org

---

Appendix B   Advanced Practice in Nephrology Nursing (page 2 of 2)

Page 2
Advanced Practice in Nephrology Nursing

l. provide leadership within the area of nephrology through consultation, clinical practice, education, and research
m. contribute to the generation of the knowledge base for nursing and specifically nephrology nursing
n. provide leadership for practice changes
o. provide leadership for nephrology nursing to be an integral part of disease management proposals
p. contribute to the advancement of the profession as a whole

• Certification of the advanced practice nurse as a clinical nurse specialist or nurse practitioner is a method to recognize competence by the profession. Certification at the advanced practice level requires a graduate degree from an accredited program that provides both the necessary didactic and clinical experiences in the area of certification.

• The advanced practice nurse in nephrology nursing refers exclusively to those caring for patients. The clinical role is central to the advanced practice nurse. Nurses with graduate degrees may hold a variety of positions including, but not limited to, management, research, education, case management, and quality management. The advanced practice nurse works collaboratively with these professionals to provide quality care.

Suggested reading list:

American Nurses Association (ANA) (2008). Guide to the code of ethics for nurses: interpretation and application. Washington, DC: Fowler, Marsha D. M., PhD, MDiv, MS, RN, FAAN, Editor

American Nephrology Nurses' Association (ANNA) (2008). Scope and Standards of Advanced Practice in Nephrology Nursing. Pitman, NJ: Brooks, Deborah H., MSN, APRN, C, CNN CNN-NP, Editor

Pearson Report (Feb 2009) The American Journal of Nurse Practitioners. (www.webnp.net).

Adopted by the American Nephrology Nurses' Association
Board of Directors
March 1997
Revised: November 1997
Revised: January 2003
Revised: July 2003
Revised: April 2005
Reaffirmed: March 2007
Revised: September 2007
Reaffirmed: February 2009

ANNA Position Statements are reviewed and reaffirmed biennially.

ANNA National Office   East Holly Avenue, Box 56   Pitman, NJ 08071-0056
Phone: 888-600-ANNA (2662) or 856-256-2320   **Fax**: 856-589-7463   **Email**: anna@ajj.com   **Website**: http://www.annanurse.org

Appendix C Certification in Nephrology Nursing (page 1 of 2)

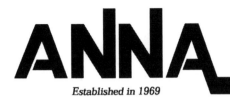

Position Statement

American Nephrology Nurses' Association

Established in 1969

Certification in Nephrology Nursing

The American Nephrology Nurses' Association (ANNA) recognizes nephrology nursing practice as a distinct nursing specialty. As such, ANNA identifies certification as one essential component to internal management of the profession. ANNA also recognizes that certification assists in protecting the public from unsafe and incompetent caregivers, gives consumers more choices in seeking health care providers, distinguishes among levels of care, and may give certified individuals a competitive advantage *(Cary, 2001.)* In order to assure public protection, ANNA recognizes and endorses nephrology nursing credentials conferred by certifying bodies that base their examinations on a periodic assessment of nephrology nursing practice via practice analyses and submit their processes to external peer review. ANNA recognizes certification at all levels.

It is the position of ANNA that:
- Certification is an essential component of specialty nursing practice
- Certification must be designed to protect the public from unsafe and incompetent caregivers
- The association will recognize and endorse certification credentials in which:
  - The examination is based on periodic practice analysis surveys.
  - The credentialing body submits to an external peer review process, ensuring the validity and integrity of the certification credential
- Certification is encouraged for all levels of nephrology nursing practice

Background and Rationale
ANNA identifies certification as an essential component of the model of nephrology nursing specialty practice (Jordan, 1993). While recognizing the need for autonomy of the certification body (ANNA, 2001), ANNA, as the professional association for the specialty, has an inherent interest in the certification of nurses practicing in the specialty. Parker (1998) identified the conferring of a standardized credential as an important means of internal management of specialty nursing practice. The American Nurses Association (1979) has identified that the main objective of certification in nursing is to assure that the public receives quality-nursing care and is safe from incompetent caregivers. Other benefits of certification may include quality care and patient satisfaction, professional recognition, financial compensation, career advancement, staff retention, personal growth, self-confidence and professional autonomy (Cary, 2001).

The need to protect the public demands the credential reflect actual practice and allow the public to infer the qualifications of the credentialed provider (Joel, 1989, Styles, 1989) Basing the test blueprint on periodic assessment of current practice via practice analysis surveys provides confidence that the examination reflects current practice. ANNA also recognizes that nursing practice has many levels: novice, advanced beginner, competent, proficient, and expert (Benner, 1984). Practice analysis supported examinations may test at any of these levels. The integrity and reliability of the examination and the entire credentialing process is strengthened by external peer review. External peer review strengthens the validity and integrity of the exam by setting standards for test construction and validity, test administration, candidate eligibility, scoring and recertification (ABNS, 1997).

ANNA National Office   East Holly Avenue, Box 56   Pitman, NJ 08071-0056
Phone: 888-600-ANNA (2662) or 856-256-2320   **Fax**: 856-589-7463   **Email**: anna@ajj.com   **Website**: http://www.annanurse.org

Appendix C Certification in Nephrology Nursing (page 2 of 2)

Page 2
Certification in Nephrology Nursing

References

American Board of Nursing Specialties. (1997). *Application for approval: Standards, rationale, criteria, required documentation.* Washington, DC: Author.

American Nephrology Nurses Association. (2001) *Position Statement on the Autonomy of the NNCC.* Pitman, NJ: Author.

American Nurses Association. The study of credentialing in nursing: a new approach. Kansas City, MO: Author, 1979.

Benner, P. (1984). *From Novice to Expert: Excellence and Power in Clinical Nursing.* Menlo Park, CA: Addison Wesley.

Cary, A.H. (2001). Certified registered nurses: Results of the study of the certified workforce. *American Journal of Nursing 101* (1), 44-51.

Joel, L. (1989). In search of a rational future for certification. *American Nurse, 21*(10).

Jordan, PJ (1993). *Nephrology Nursing: A guide to professional development.* Pitman, NJ: American Nephrology Nurses Association

Parker, J (1998) Nephrology nursing as a specialty. In: Parker, J (ed) *Contemporary Nephrology Nursing.* Pitman, NJ: American Nephrology Nurses Association.

Styles, M (1989) *On specialization in nursing: Towards a new empowerment.* Kansas City, MO: American Nurses Foundation, Inc

Adopted by the American Nephrology Nurses' Association
Board of Directors
March 2003
Reaffirmed: November 2003
Reaffirmed: April 2005
Reaffirmed: February 2008

Appendix D ANNA Health Policy Statement (page 1 of 6)

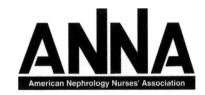

HEALTH POLICY STATEMENT

PREAMBLE

The American Nephrology Nurses' Association (ANNA) is a national organization of registered nurses practicing in nephrology, which includes but is not limited to hemodialysis and peritoneal dialysis therapies, Chronic Kidney Disease (CKD), transplantation and continuous renal replacement therapies. ANNA members are involved in the supervision and delivery of care to children and adults who have or are at risk of kidney disease. ANNA supports the interdisciplinary approach to health care and believes that registered nurses must be major participants in the planning, delivery and evaluation of that care.

As a professional organization, ANNA has the obligation to set and update standards of patient care, educate practitioners, stimulate research and disseminate findings, promote interdisciplinary communication and cooperation, and address issues that may impact the practice of nephrology nursing.

This Health Policy Statement represents the ANNA viewpoint on major public policy issues relevant to the treatment of individuals with kidney disease and the practice of professional nephrology nursing. This document serves to give the Association direction as legislative and regulatory issues are addressed on local, state and national levels. This document has been developed based on a comprehensive review of current issues and with input from ANNA members and leaders.

NURSING

1. ANNA is committed to assuring and protecting access to professional nursing care delivered by highly educated, well-trained, and experienced registered nurses for individuals with kidney disease.

2. ANNA believes that a baccalaureate degree in nursing is the minimum requirement for entry into professional nursing practice.

3. ANNA supports the promotion of the nurse's role in health policy advocacy through educational efforts, grassroots outreach, and other activities that seek to promote the health and well being of individuals, families, and communities affected by real or potential kidney disease.

4. ANNA supports the inclusion of registered nurses in policy development at all levels of government and on all boards, commissions, expert panels, task forces and other groups setting policies and standards that affect nursing practice, the Medicare End Stage Renal Disease (ESRD) program, and its beneficiaries.

5. ANNA supports efforts to resolve the nursing shortage, including measures to assure appropriate funding to address the shortage of nursing faculty and the availability of nursing mentors for new graduates and inexperienced nurses.

Appendix D ANNA Health Policy Statement (page 2 of 6)

6. Congruent with the Centers for Medicare and Medicaid (CMS), ANNA believes that registered nurses experienced in dialytic therapy must be present to provide assessment and direct supervision of patient care activities and unlicensed personnel during dialysis treatments.

7. ANNA believes that a registered nurse must be actively involved in determining staffing requirements in facilities providing care to patients with kidney disease, and that these requirements should include consideration of patient condition and specific medical and/or psychosocial needs.

8. ANNA believes that care of patients with kidney disease is provided effectively and responsibly by registered nurses and unlicensed assistive personnel in ratios that are based on patient needs and acuity. Further, the use of advanced practice registered nurses in the management of patients with kidney disease can result in cost efficient high quality care, benefiting the health care delivery system in general, and the Medicare ESRD program in particular. ANNA supports the recognition of compensation for advanced practice registered nurses by all payers – public and private.

9. Congruent with the Medicare Improvements for Patients and Providers Act of 2008 (MIPPA), the Association believes that a sound education program is necessary to develop, maintain, and augment clinical and technical competence. ANNA believes that all licensed patient care personnel must complete a standardized nephrology education program reflecting the ANNA *Nephrology Nursing Standards of Care and Guidelines for Practice*.

10. ANNA endorses the certification of qualified nephrology nurses as defined by the Nephrology Nursing Certification Commission and continuing certification to refine the knowledge of nurses providing care to individuals in all stages and types of kidney disease across the life span.

11. ANNA supports a nurse's right to refuse to perform an act or take an assignment that in the nurse's judgment is not safe or is not within that nurse's skill, experience, qualifications or capability.

12. In accordance with our commitment to compassionate end-of-life care, ANNA believes that nurses should not participate in assisted suicide or active euthanasia and that such acts are in direct violation of the American Nurses Association (ANA) Code for Nurses with Interpretive Statements and the ethical traditions of the profession (ANA, 2001). ANNA supports the ANA statement which asserts that, "Nurses individually and collectively have an obligation to provide comprehensive and compassionate end-of-life care which includes the promotion of comfort and the relief of pain and, at times, foregoing life-sustaining treatment." ANNA acknowledges that refusal to participate in assisted suicide or euthanasia does not constitute abandonment of patients.

13. ANNA believes that nephrology nurses should continue to advocate policies and programs that promote and ensure health care environments that provide humane and dignified patient-centered care. The Association supports continued dialogue, education, and research on end-of-life issues and appropriate decision-making related to discontinuation of or withdrawal from dialysis treatment. ANNA has endorsed the *Clinical Practice Guideline on Shared Decision-Making in the Appropriate Initiation and Withdrawal from Dialysis* (February 2000), published by the Renal Physicians Association and the American Society of Nephrology.

Appendix D ANNA Health Policy Statement (page 3 of 6)

14. ANNA believes health care personnel must be protected from occupational and environmental health hazards related to dialytic therapy and that standards for safety and protective measures should be developed, identified, and implemented.

15. ANNA believes that any efforts to detect or test for substance abuse or communicable diseases must be consistent with good medical practice and shall not violate the individual's civil rights.

16. ANNA supports the state Boards of Nursing efforts to implement multistate licensure for health professionals through expansion of the interstate compact.

17. ANNA supports improved provision of and access to telehealth services, both distance learning for professionals and patients as well as treatment and home monitoring of patients with chronic diseases for Medicare and Medicaid beneficiaries. We support not only the concept of telehealth but also the development of methods to reimburse providers in rural or underserved areas for these services.

18. ANNA endorses the Nursing Organizations Alliance (NOA) "Principles and Elements of a Healthful Practice/Work Environment" (July 2005), and the American Association of Critical Care Nurses (AACN) Standards for Establishing and Sustaining Health Work Environment (2005).

ELEMENTS OF CARE

1. ANNA believes the practice of nephrology nursing is directed toward assessing and treating the health needs of individuals and their families who are experiencing the real or threatened impact of compromised kidney function, and/or acute or chronic kidney disease. This practice includes a commitment to help each individual and his/her significant others achieve an optimal level of functioning. Toward this end, nephrology nurses must establish high standards of patient care that are routinely updated.

2. ANNA believes that appropriate, quality treatment must be available to all individuals with kidney disease and other disease processes that require replacement therapies. ANNA supports providing these individuals with complete and accurate information about all alternative forms of therapy, including the associated risks and benefits, without regard for their cost. The Association believes that these individuals and their significant others must be encouraged and allowed to be active participants in this decision-making process.

3. ANNA supports legislative, regulatory, and programmatic efforts that promote prevention and management of chronic kidney disease, including early diagnosis, education and proactive creation of native fistulae for dialysis. ANNA is fully committed to working with Congress, CMS, and the larger kidney community to implement the education and prevention provisions of the MIPPA legislation. ANNA supports nephrology nursing participation in the Fistula First Initiative on the state and federal level.

4. In order to achieve the goal of optimal rehabilitation, ANNA believes individuals must assume as much responsibility for their overall care as their physical and mental limits allow. ANNA supports all home and self-dialysis modalities, with training and supervision of persons choosing these modalities being under the direction of a qualified registered nurse. Additionally, ANNA supports research into barriers to home dialysis and access to balanced education for people with kidney disease that includes home therapy as a treatment option. Reducing barriers to self-care may assist in increasing access to

Appendix D   ANNA Health Policy Statement (page 4 of 6)

Health Policy Statement
Page 4

dialysis care in light of predictions that people requiring dialysis in the next two decades is expected to double in number.

5. ANNA supports the dialysis payment reforms within the MIPPA law and will continue to play an active role in the implementation of theses changes. ANNA supports any efforts to allow flexibility for the provision of daily or more frequent dialysis, and any other safe and effective emerging treatment modalities for chronic kidney disease, including incentives for patient self-management.

6. ANNA believes that all individuals including health care providers must be protected from the possible threat of communicable diseases related to dialysis, transplantation, and other extracorporeal therapies, and that access to testing for such diseases should be available to all patients and health care providers. ANNA endorses the vaccination of all patients against Hepatitis B, pneumonia, and influenza and the Centers for Disease Control and Prevention (CDC) vaccination recommendations for nephrology staff.

7. ANNA supports legislative, regulatory, and programmatic efforts that promote disaster preparedness and early identification, triage, and evacuation if necessary, of patients requiring kidney replacement therapy during disaster situations.

TRANSPLANTATION

1. ANNA supports public and private sector efforts that promote organ donation and increase transplantation. The Association believes this can be accomplished by:

    a. Continued support for educational programs for the public and for health professionals addressing the shortage of donor organs and the appropriate identification of potential donors;

    b. Continued support for the federally funded Organ Procurement and Transplantation Network and the Scientific Registry;

    c. Implementation of uniform state laws regarding organ donation, procurement, and transplantation:

        i. Amend the Anatomical Gift Act to support that a desire to donate or not to donate expressed in any form (a donor card, driver's license check-off, placement of name on a registry, or verbal statement) cannot be revoked by the next of kin. (This would prohibit approaching families when there is clear evidence that the individual did not want to donate);

        ii. Amend the Anatomical Gift Act to facilitate Medical Examiner/ Coroner consent for 'John Doe' donations following a diligent search for identification and legal next of kin;

        iii. Include organ/tissue donation language in all legislative and regulatory proposals related to advance directives, living wills, and durable powers of attorney; and

        iv. Support of state registries for persons wishing to donate organs at the time of their death and federal funding for these registries.

    d. Continued federal support of transplant activities including medical research and coverage of immunosuppressive drug therapy and legislative initiatives to extend immunosuppressive drug coverage for the life of the transplanted organ(s);

    e. Educate insurers and other payers regarding the success and cost effectiveness of organ transplantation for their members and encourage activities that decrease actual or perceived barriers to transplantation;

Appendix D ANNA Health Policy Statement (page 5 of 6)

    f. Removal of financial disincentives to live organ donation including funding for transportation and lost income;

    g. Studies to review the ethical implications of proposals to increase living non-related donation that may disproportionately affect certain populations; and

    h. Support for research into the use of financial incentives for deceased donors as a potential mechanism to increase organ donation.

2. ANNA opposes coercive behavior in the solicitation of organs for transplantation and live donation when the donor's decision is based primarily on financial gain.

ESRD PROGRAM MANAGEMENT

1. ANNA supports ESRD payment reforms that support delivery of care that is consistent with both the standards of professional nephrology nursing established by ANNA, and current professionally accepted clinical practice guidelines and standards established by the renal professional community.

2. ANNA believes that patients with CKD should have access to education and support services and clinical care that may improve their kidney function, delay the progression of their disease, or improve their health status and readiness for the initiation of end stage renal disease therapies.

3. ANNA supports amending Title XIX of the Social Security Act (Medicaid) to include dialysis as a mandatory service in state Medicaid programs.

4. ANNA believes that oversight of ESRD facilities should be an ongoing, collaborative effort by CMS and its contractors, including state agencies and renal Network organizations. Members of the on-site survey team should be knowledgeable about the various aspects of the delivery of care to individuals with kidney disease.

5. ANNA supports the timely inspection and approval of ESRD facilities that will increase patient's access to care.

MANAGED CARE AND COMMERCIAL HEALTH PLANS AND THE ESRD POPULATION

ANNA believes that all health plans must:

1. Develop a process to ensure access of members diagnosed with CKD or ESRD to relevant specialists.

2. Develop a protocol or incentives for encouraging screening members for kidney disease and early referral of those members to nephrologists for evaluation and interventions.

3. Have a mechanism for providing access for members with ESRD to dialysis and transplant providers that are geographically accessible, whose outcomes and waiting times are known to meet acceptable national standards and averages, and that are able to provide all forms of dialytic therapy currently available, including peritoneal dialysis, home dialysis, and a dialysis schedule that conforms with the members' employment or other rehabilitation needs.

4. Involve nephrology professionals and/or utilize available clinical practice guidelines in the development of care delivery models for members with CKD.

Appendix D   ANNA Health Policy Statement (page 6 of 6)

5.   Provide case management services that collaborate with nephrology providers for a comprehensive, patient centered plan of care that provides optimal kidney replacement therapy and palliative care when necessary.

6.   Develop mechanisms to ensure the inclusion of members with ESRD in the ESRD Network programs and the United States Renal Data System (USRDS) database.

7.   ANNA believes that all health plans must conduct periodic evaluations of all contractors (e.g. dialysis facilities and transplant programs) providing care to members with end-stage renal disease.

8.   Provide coverage for dialysis services for members who travel outside the health plan's normal coverage area.

9.   Provide coverage for immunosuppressive agents for all transplant recipients for the duration of the transplant.

10.   Provide coverage for hospice care.

11.   Not discriminate in any way against a member on the basis of a diagnosis of ESRD or a condition that leads to chronic kidney disease.

Adopted by the American Nephrology Nurses' Association Board of Directors in March 1997
Revised and/or reaffirmed annually from 1998-2009
Most recently revised: February 2010

The Health Policy Statement is reviewed and reaffirmed annually.

Appendix E Principles and Elements of a Healthful Practice/Work Environment

Principles and Elements of a Healthful Practice/Work Environment

The Nursing Organizations Alliance believes that a healthful practice/work environment is supported by the presence of the following elements:

1. **Collaborative Practice Culture**

   Respectful collegial communication & behavior
   Team orientation
   Presence of trust
   Respect for diversity

2. **Communication Rich Culture**

   Clear and respectful
   Open and trusting

3. **A Culture of Accountability**

   Role expectations are clearly defined
   Everyone is accountable

4. **The Presence of Adequate Numbers of Qualified Nurses**

   Ability to provide quality care to meet client/patient's needs
   Work/home life balance

5. **The Presence of Expert, Competent, Credible, Visible Leadership**

   Serve as an advocate for nursing practice
   Support shared decision making
   Allocate resources to support nursing

6. **Shared Decision Making at All Levels**

   Nurses participate in system, organizational, and process decisions
   Formal structure exists to support shared decision making
   Nurses have control over their practice

7. **The Encouragement of Professional Practice & Continued Growth/Development**

   Continuing education/certification is supported/encouraged
   Participation in professional association encouraged
   An information rich environment is supported

8. **Recognition of the Value of Nursing's Contribution**

   Reward and pay for performance
   Career mobility and expansion

9. **Recognition by Nurses for Their Meaningful Contribution to Practice**

   These nine elements will be fostered and promoted, as best fits, into the work of individual member organizations of the Alliance.

American Organization of Nurse Executives
~2004~

Appendix F Reference Card (page 1 of 2)

Reference Card From the

Seventh Report of the Joint National Committee on Prevention, Detection, Evaluation, and Treatment of High Blood Pressure (JNC 7)

EVALUATION

Classification of Blood Pressure (BP)*

Category	SBP mmHg		DBP mmHg
Normal	<120	and	<80
Prehypertension	120–139	or	80–89
Hypertension, Stage 1	140–159	or	90–99
Hypertension, Stage 2	□160	or	□100

* See Blood Pressure Measurement Techniques (reverse side)
Key: SBP = systolic blood pressure DBP = diastolic blood pressure

Diagnostic Workup of Hypertension

- Assess risk factors and comorbidities.
- Reveal identifiable causes of hypertension.
- Assess presence of target organ damage.
- Conduct history and physical examination.
- Obtain laboratory tests: urinalysis, blood glucose, hematocrit and lipid panel, serum potassium, creatinine, and calcium. Optional: urinary albumin/creatinine ratio.
- Obtain electrocardiogram .

Assess for Major Cardiovascular Disease (CVD) Risk Factors

- Hypertension
- Obesity (body mass index >_30 kg/m²)
- Dyslipidemia
- Diabetes mellitus
- Cigarette smoking
- Physical inactivity
- Microalbuminuria, estimated glomerular filtration rate <60 mL/min
- Age (>55 for men, >65 for women)
- Family history of premature CVD (men age <55, women age <65)

Assess for Identifiable Causes of Hypertension

- Sleep apnea
- Drug induced/related
- Chronic kidney disease
- Primary aldosteronism
- Renovascular disease
- Cushing's syndrome or steroid therapy
- Pheochromocytoma
- Coarctation of aorta
- Thyroid/parathyroid disease

U.S. DEPARTMENT OF HEALTH AND HUMAN SERVICES
National Institutes of Health
National Heart, Lung, and Blood Institute

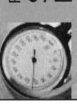

TREATMENT

Principles of Hypertension Treatment

- Treat to BP <140/90 mmHg or BP <130/80 mmHg in patients with diabetes or chronic kidney dise ise.
- Majority of patients will require two medications to reach goal.

Algorithm for Treatment o Hypertension

Lifestyle Modifications

↓

Not at Goal Blood Pressure (<140/90 mmHg)
(<130/80 mmHg for patients with diabetes or chronic kidney disease)
See Strategies for Improving Adherence to Therapy

↓

Initial Drug Choices

Without Compelling Indications

Stage 1 Hypertension (SBP 140–159 or DBP 90–99 mmHg)

Thiazide-type diuretics for most. May consider ACEI, ARB, BB, CCB, or combination.

Stage 2 Hypertension (SBP ≥160 or DBP ≥100 mmHg)

2-drug combination for most (usually thiazide-type diuretic and ACEI, or ARB, or BB, or CCB).

With Compelling Indications

Drug(s) for the compelling indications See Compelling Indications for Individual Drug Classes

Other antihypertensive drugs (diuretics, ACEI, ARB, BB, CCB) as needed.

↓

Not at Goal Blood Pressure

Optimize dosages or add additional drugs until goal blood pressure is achieved. Consider consultation with hypertension specialist.
See Strategies for Improving Adherence to Therapy

Appendix F   Reference Card (page 2 of 2)

Blood Pressure Measurement Techniques

Method	Notes
In-office	Two readings, 5 minutes apart, sitting in chair. Confirm elevated reading in contralateral arm.
Ambulatory BP monitoring	Indicated for evaluation of "white coat hypertension." Absence of 10–20 percent BP decrease during sleep may indicate increased CVD risk.
Patient self-check	Provides information on response to therapy. May help improve adherence to therapy and is useful for evaluating "white coat hypertension."

Causes of Resistant Hypertension

- Improper BP measurement
- Excess sodium intake
- Inadequate diuretic therapy
- Medication
  - Inadequate doses
  - Drug actions and interactions (e.g., nonsteroidal anti-inflammatory drugs (NSAIDs), illicit drugs, sympathomimetics, oral contraceptives)
  - Over-the-counter (OTC) drugs and herbal supplements
- Excess alcohol intake
- Identifiable causes of hypertension (see reverse side)

Compelling Indications for Individual Drug Classes

Compelling Indication	Initial Therapy Options
Heart failure	THIAZ, BB, ACEI, ARB, ALDO ANT
Post myocardial infarction	BB, ACEI, ALDO ANT
High CVD risk	THIAZ, BB, ACEI, CCB
Diabetes	THIAZ, BB, ACEI, ARB, CCB
Chronic kidney disease	ACEI, ARB
Recurrent stroke prevention	THIAZ, ACEI

Key: THIAZ = thiazide diuretic, ACEI= angiotensin converting enzyme inhibitor, ARB = angiotensin receptor blocker, BB = beta blocker, CCB = calcium channel blocker, ALDO ANT = aldosterone antagonist

Strategies for Improving Adherence to Therapy

- Clinician empathy increases patient trust, motivation, and adherence to therapy.
- Physicians should consider their patients' cultural beliefs and individual attitudes in formulating therapy.

Principles of Lifestyle Modification

- Encourage healthy lifestyles for all individuals.
- Prescribe lifestyle modifications for all patients with prehypertension and hypertension.
- Components of lifestyle modifications include weight reduction, DASH eating plan, dietary sodium reduction, aerobic physical activity, and moderation of alcohol consumption.

Lifestyle Modification Recommendations

Modification	Recommendation	Avg. SBP Reduction Range†
Weight reduction	Maintain normal body weight (body mass index 18.5–24.9 kg/m²).	5–20 mmHg/10 kg
DASH eating plan	Adopt a diet rich in fruits, vegetables, and lowfat dairy products with reduced content of saturated and total fat.	8–14 mmHg
Dietary sodium reduction	Reduce dietary sodium intake to ≤100 mmol per day (2.4 g sodium or 6 g sodium chloride).	2–8 mmHg
Aerobic physical activity	Regular aerobic physical activity (e.g., brisk walking) at least 30 minutes per day, most days of the week.	4–9 mmHg
Moderation of alcohol consumption	Men: limit to ≤2 drinks* per day. Women and lighter weight persons: limit to ≤1 drink* per day.	2–4 mmHg

* 1 drink = 1/2 oz or 15 mL ethanol (e.g., 12 oz beer, 5 oz wine, 1.5 oz 80-proof whiskey).
† Effects are dose and time dependent.

U.S. DEPARTMENT OF HEALTH AND HUMAN SERVICES
National Institutes of Health
National Heart, Lung, and Blood Institute
National High Blood Pressure Education Program

NIH Publication No. 03-5231
May 2003

The National High Blood Pressure Education Program is coordinated by the National Heart, Lung, and Blood Institute (NHLBI) at the National Institutes of Health. Copies of the JNC 7 Report are available on the NHLBI Web site at   http//www.nhlbi.nih.gov   or from the NHLBI Health Information Center, P.O. Box 30105, Bethesda, MD 20824-0105; Phone: 301-592-8573 or 240-629-3255 (TTY); Fax: 301-592-8563.